Your Orgasmic Pregnancy

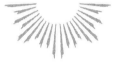

ORDERING
Trade bookstores in the U.S. and Canada please contact:

Publishers Group West
1700 Fourth Street, Berkeley CA 94710
Phone: (800) 788-3123   Fax: (800) 351-5073

Hunter House books are available at bulk discounts
for textbook course adoptions; to qualifying community, health-care,
and government organizations; and for special promotions and fund-raising.
For details please contact:

Special Sales Department
Hunter House Inc., PO Box 2914, Alameda CA 94501-0914
Phone: (510) 865-5282   Fax: (510) 865-4295
E-mail: ordering@hunterhouse.com

Individuals can order our books from most bookstores,
by calling **(800) 266-5592**, or from our website at
www.hunterhouse.com

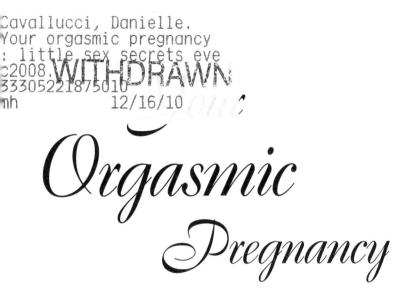

Your Orgasmic Pregnancy

Little Sex Secrets Every Hot Mama Should Know

DANIELLE CAVALLUCCI

and

YVONNE K. FULBRIGHT, PhD

Hunter House
PUBLISHERS

Hunter House Inc., Publishers
PO Box 2914
Alameda CA 94501-0914

LIBRARY OF CONGRESS CATALOGING-IN-PUBLICATION DATA
Cavallucci, Danielle.
Your orgasmic pregnancy : little sex secrets every hot mama should know /
Danielle Cavallucci and Yvonne K. Fulbright.
p. cm.
Includes bibliographical references and index.
ISBN-13: 978-0-89793-501-2 (pbk.)
ISBN-10: 0-89793-501-2 (pbk.)
1. Pregnant women—Sexual behavior.   2. Pregnant women—Health and hygiene.
3. Sensuality.   I. Fulbright, Yvonne K.   II. Title.
RG525.C383 2008
618.2—dc22   2007048897

PROJECT CREDITS

Cover Design: Brian Dittmar Graphic Design
Book Production: John McKercher
Illustrator: Joshua McKenney
Developmental and Copy Editor:
Kelley Blewster
Proofreader: John David Marion
Indexer: Yvonne K. Fulbright
Acquisitions Editor: Jeanne Brondino
Editor: Alexandra Mummery

Senior Marketing Associate: Reina Santana
Rights Coordinator: Candace Groskreutz
Production Assistant: Amy Hagelin
Customer Service Manager:
Christina Sverdrup
Order Fulfillment: Washul Lakdhon
Administrator: Theresa Nelson
Computer Support: Peter Eichelberger
Publisher: Kiran S. Rana

Printed and Bound by Bang Printing, Brainerd, Minnesota

Manufactured in the United States of America

9 8 7 6 5 4 3 2 1   First Edition   08 09 10 11 12

Contents

List of Illustrations

Acknowledgments

We extend our deepest, most heartfelt thanks to the inspired and generous souls who made this book possible.

First and foremost, our appreciation goes to all of the women and men, quoted and not, whose stories and support contributed to the completion of this book. We thank each of you dynamic and sexy women, and your supportive partners, who rallied behind our cause from start to finish and believed not only that we could, but that we should.

To the Hunter House team—publisher Kiran Rana, acquisitions editor Jeanne Brondino, editor Alex Mummery, editor Kelley Blewster, and marketing associate Reina Santana. We are deeply moved by your belief in our vision.

To our families for their love and support, particularly Danielle's grandmother, Gisela Johnson, and Yvonne's parents, Charles G. Fulbright and Ósk Lárusdóttir Fulbright.

To Bryson Coles at Snowday Designs for a sensual website and all of his tireless work perfecting it.

To Amanda Meulenberg, MD, for her support, great input, and invaluable expertise in making sure that all of our medical information was good to go.

To Paula D. Atkinson for her yoga expertise and wonderful energy.

To John O'Connor for his expertise in massage therapy and continued support of our Sensual Fusion quest.

To Stephen Gamboa, MD, for his feedback, wisdom, and support.

And last, but certainly not least, to our illustrator, Joshua McKenney, for the wonderful illustrations that complement this work.

Yikes!
The Goddess
Is with Child

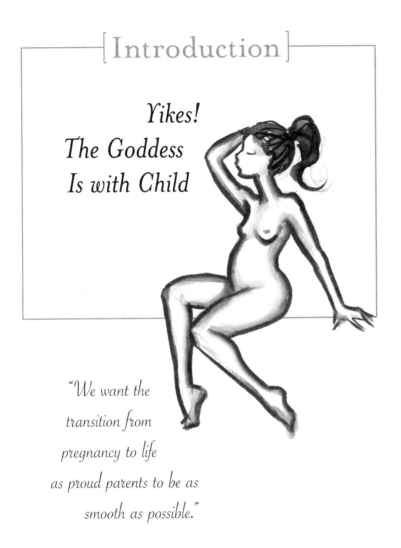

"We want the
transition from
pregnancy to life
as proud parents to be as
smooth as possible."

*C*ongratulations, Hot Mama in the making! By opening this book you have taken the first step toward owning your body, your intimacy potential, and your sexuality during your pregnancy and beyond. We, your Hot Mama mentors, look forward to helping you make the most of this profound, life-altering experience that will shape and enhance you as a sexual being. Rejecting the notion that pregnant women cannot or should not be sexpots, we aim to ensure that the next nine-plus months don't turn into one long sexual sabbatical for you, but rather are jam-packed with some of the best lovemaking experiences you have ever known. We want you to feel like the sex kitten you are, and to believe that, with a little advice and female-to-female empowerment, it *is* possible for any woman to feel downright sexually primed while in the family way.

ॐ I Am Sexy, Hear Me Roar!

You may have noticed that Hot Mamas have been quite the hot topic lately. Preggies everywhere are demanding that their presence be acknowledged. So why is the woman with child suddenly so irresistible? Modern societies are finally celebrating the fact that pregnancy is the ultimate expression of sexual union and not some immaculate conception. The merging of two beings, resulting in a life-form, is being hailed not only as miraculous, but also as a clear tribute to the power of sexual attraction, to the intermingling of spirits, and to the awe-inspiring role Mother Nature has bestowed upon women. The prevailing attitude, which is at the heart of this book (and is long overdue, in our opinions), has become: Why not embrace and celebrate the fact that pregnancy is, at its very essence, a sexual experience? And who better to stand up for women everywhere in their quest to become sexually fulfilled than an expectant tigress shouting, "I am sexual, hear me roar!"

No longer must you choose between being sexy or being maternal—you can be both! This book aims to help you unleash your deepest sensual self by presenting handy pointers, frank information, and academic research.

Sure, we realize that staying sexy may be the farthest thing from a newly pregnant woman's mind. Amid the chaos and elation surrounding the discovery that you are expecting, sex may drop far down on a couple's list of priorities, especially in light of the planning and preparation required for a newborn. We're here to gently remind you that your sex life still matters—indeed, that it needs to take precedence at this important juncture. We want to encourage pregnant women to take a look, sooner than later, at their sexuality and lovemaking. After all, pregnancy is among the most significant events in your life and in your relationship. We want you to embrace the fact that pregnancy and motherhood can cause you, and your partner, to feel more sensual than ever.

Need further persuading? Know that building your pregnancy on a sexy, confident foundation is as important to your parenting skills as it is to your partnership. A fulfilled Hot Mama is a happy mother, which makes for a happy child. Believe it or not, your sex life can indirectly have lasting effects on the outcome of your child's life. And if that's not incentive enough to make you want to read up on the subject, we don't know what is!

🐾 Finding Your Sensual Grail

Regardless of whether you find yourself howling in heat, entertaining all-consuming sexual fantasies, or simply convinced that intimacy should be a top priority during pregnancy, we know how challenging it can be to get accurate and pertinent information on this topic. As you may have already discovered, most books on pregnancy devote a mere page or two to the subject of pregnant sex, and the bit of material that is available is typically devoted to the technical aspects of the act. Few resources explore the "un-mommy-like" topics of increased desire, more intense orgasm, and "unconventional" sex play, especially the way we do in this book. Until now, you may have found yourself a bit discouraged, wondering whether you're the only Hot Mama on the planet who wants to get down and dirty.

Rest assured that you are not alone. You are in the company of thousands of women who cherish the sensual beauty of pregnancy and are discovering that a Hot Mama's body in all its stages, including postbirth, can be a wonderfully sensual thing. Women like you are our inspiration for writing this book.

Some of the topics we've addressed include:

* ❖ how to feel sexy, desirable, and luscious throughout your pregnancy and beyond

* ❖ embracing the pregnancy-related surge in libido and sexual fantasizing

* ❖ understanding the biological and bodily changes impacting your sex life

✻ exploring—and exploiting—your orgasmic potential

✻ dealing with the "third party" relationship between you, your partner, and your babe (both before birth and after)

✻ how to feel fresh, energized, and ready for intimate moments

✻ maintaining intimate activity at every stage of pregnancy, including those times when intercourse is off-limits

✻ sexual positions suitable for preggies and their partners

✻ postpartum intimacy

✻ the latest research on sexuality and intimacy during and after pregnancy

✻ allowing yourself to explore sexual behaviors often considered naughty no-no's for pregnant women

✻ how to communicate your sexual needs and concerns to your health-care provider and other confidants

✻ staying in sync with your partner

✻ answers to taboo questions

✻ making the most of pregnancy's unique opportunities to improve and expand your sex life

We're here to help you define what sort of sexy mama you are and want to become so that you can reap the erotic rewards of pregnancy. *Your Orgasmic Pregnancy* presents a candid, spirited, and fearless discussion devoted solely to celebrating the sex goddess in all her pregnant majesty, and it seeks to make a significant and positive impact on your quality of life, and that of your partner and babe.

🐾 Meet Your Sex Coaches

When we announced this book we received many e-mails of support and thanks, which reinforced our belief that we had hit upon an extremely important issue. Many women gushed about the opportunity to speak frankly on a topic that few understand and even fewer talk about in depth. We realized that we were not simply advocating for better sex and relationships, but were also empowering women everywhere, pregnant or not. On the following pages you will find a blend of Danielle's firsthand experience as a pregnant woman and Yvonne's expertise in sexuality and relationships. You will also read real-life stories from other women, as well as from a few men, who felt inspired to share their experiences in the hopes of encouraging others.

After we met at a party in New York City in 2002, your Hot Mama mentors became fast friends. We instantly recognized our overlapping interest in topics related to sexuality and our mutual desire to liberate lovers worldwide. Danielle works in the film industry, and also as a life coach and certified nutrition and fitness trainer. Yvonne has worked for more than a decade as a sexuality coach, educator, and sexologist. We promised to someday work together on a project, and it was Danielle's pregnancy in 2005—especially her search for information on maintaining her sex life and her feelings of loving connectedness with her partner during pregnancy—that motivated us to write this book. We knew it was time to collaborate on a work that would cultivate better, more loving, and more sexually satisfying relationships for expectant couples. *Your Orgasmic Pregnancy: Little Sex Secrets Every Hot Mama Should Know* is our first-born "pen child," and we hope you enjoy and benefit from it immensely.

☙ Getting the Most from This Book

Intended to benefit heterosexual, bisexual, and lesbian women alike, this book can be read at any stage of your pregnancy. After getting you "in the mood," we walk you through each trimester, focusing on what you're likely to experience sexually. We want the transition from pregnancy to life as proud parents to be as smooth as possible, so we wrap things up with information and tips on reclaiming your body, recharging your sex life, and staying close to your partner while juggling life with a new babe.

Whether you read the book in one sitting or over the course of your pregnancy, we recommend reading the chapters in order, especially as they relate to where you are in your pregnancy. Chapter 5, on good self-care during pregnancy, can be read at any point. It's a good idea to read the postbirth chapters before your new babe enters the world, because afterward you're going to have little time for any leisure reading (and we want the private time you do have to involve much sexier activities!).

Please feel free to share this publication with your partner and your girlfriends. Reading it together can spark eye-opening conversations that will result in greater intimacy, sexual and otherwise. Talking about these issues with your partner and other trusted confidants will deepen your interactions with them while also increasing your comfort level and confidence by getting important topics out into the open, where change and acceptance are possible.

Note the sidebars that appear throughout the book. Those titled "For Hot Mamas: What's Going on with Your Partner" highlight the fact that improved sexual intimacy is a team effort. Those titled "For Partners: How You Can Help Her" offer your partner tips on how to better support you. Commentary by OB-GYN specialist Dr. Amanda Meulenberg aims to clarify any medical-related concerns you may have about getting your groove on while pregnant.

Whether this is your first pregnancy or one of many, we hope that this book will expand your intimacy potential and equip you with excellent tips for maintaining a sizzling, passionate sex life filled with tender moments. Staying close to your partner physically, emotionally, spiritually, and sexually is necessary both for a happy, satisfying pregnancy and to expedite a seamless reconnection between the two of you after the birth. (Better yet is to avoid the need to *re*-connect at all!) We wish you, your partner, and your little one all the best.

—Your Hot Mama mentors,
Danielle and Yvonne

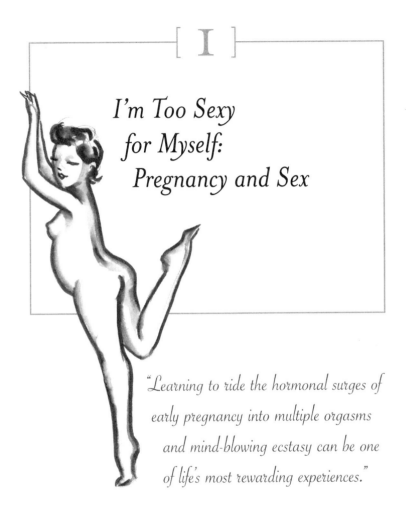

[I]

I'm Too Sexy for Myself: Pregnancy and Sex

"Learning to ride the hormonal surges of early pregnancy into multiple orgasms and mind-blowing ecstasy can be one of life's most rewarding experiences."

*C*arrying a gift created in passionate union titillated me (Danielle) no end. I was bursting with life and sensual yearnings. Daydreaming, night dreaming, feeling possessed by fantasy, pawing my partner in hopes of gaining relief from overwhelming desire—it may never have occurred to me that pregnancy wasn't "supposed to be" sexy, according to the unenlightened masses, had it not been for a few encounters with misinformation and misconceptions. TV programs and news articles chronicling the complaints of pregnant women that they or their partners had trouble finding any sexiness in pregnancy simply baffled me. Pregnant women are beautiful and exude more sexuality than at any other time in their lives. How could any woman *not* feel sensual with life budding in her belly? How could anyone else see her as anything but sexual? And how dare anyone diminish the lovefest going on between me, my partner, and my babe. We were thoroughly tickled by all of it. Aside from the absolute exhaustion of early pregnancy, which bade me to curl up and sleep eighteen of every twenty-four hours, I felt as sultry as ever. So did many of my preggie friends, and they, too, were irate at any notion that they were less than sexy.

We preggies found refuge in each another's company, disabusing one another of the fallacies surrounding our growing sensuality. We realized that, when pressed, almost every nonpreggie would fess up to loving the pregnant form. We discovered that a large number of men liked the pregnant body—both for its aesthetics and because it conveys a compelling mystique. As thirty-two-year-old Jay, a graduate student and a loving, sensual papa, eloquently says, "When you say the word 'sexy,' it has implications of the *social* stereotype of what's sexy—these false images like the flirty cheerleader or the girl on the beer commercial. A preggie isn't sexy in that way. There's something very cool and sophisticated about her. She's chic. Elegant. To me, her look implies someone who has come to grips with certain elemental things about this world—she's become part of the whole scheme of everything. And there's something so sensual about that."

This and similar comments from men we interviewed reinforced our hunch that most preggies would feel pretty good about their bodies were it not for culturally driven myths that pregnancy isn't sexy. After all, my pregnant friends and I were glowing, and everyone around us—friends, family, lovers—noticed. Think about it: Nothing is sexier than the physical proof that you've been getting it on. So it's somewhat astounding that the general consensus is that those in the family way must don the scarlet letter "A" for "asexual." It's as if society chooses to ignore how your temporary tenant took up lodging in the first place!

₷ This Isn't Your Mother's Pregnancy Manual

"My mom, grandma, and aunt haven't said a lot about sex during pregnancy, so I talk to close friends, especially those who have been pregnant," says thirty-year-old social worker Sabine, who is pregnant with her first. "What also helps is that you're seeing a lot more maternity boutiques with fashionable, hip clothes, which makes a big difference in enhancing a pregnant belly and splurging on yourself. There's a lot more emphasis on being sexy, which is exciting, compared to twenty-plus years ago, when pregnancy was more of an expected role for women. Today it's cool to be pregnant. People get excited, which creates positive energy. People like to touch you, and that's connecting. It's such a special time in everybody's life—you're creating a baby and everyone feels more bonded."

When it comes to pregnancy and sexuality, the times they are a-changin', especially among pregnant women themselves. Bold preggies everywhere are daring to own their sexuality. Witness the rise in out-of-wedlock births in the United States to an all-time high in 2006, the increasingly common phenomenon of women breastfeeding in public, and the advance in mommy-friendly activism and legislation. Add to this the fact that Hot Mama maternity wear is everywhere, along with preggie lingerie, erotica, and even porn, and you can see that the sexy preggie icon is making her mark. And to its credit, the public is starting to catch on once again.

Many millennia ago, women, especially pregnant ones, were idolized. Paleolithic cave-wall paintings dating from forty thousand to ten thousand years ago depict triangles, which are believed to be symbols of the vagina. Historians believe that early humans honored pregnant women because procreation was such a mystery. Ancient peoples were astounded by the fact that women could bloom with big belly and breasts (and likely, in some cases, a voracious sex drive)—and eventually pop out a new life.

🦋 Sex Fears and Myths

We know what you're thinking. The Hot Mama movement sounds great—thank God it's catching on during *my* pregnancy! You can count me in *but* there are those circumstances that can legitimately bench a preggie. Am I truly safe being a seductress, especially in the sack?

There are many misperceptions about sex during pregnancy that can understandably worry expectant parents. Lots of Hot Mamas have concerns and questions about the whole intimacy equation—for example, when, where, how, and how much? —which, left unidentified and unanswered, can lead to sexual challenges. So let's address these first:

The most common sexual concern for both partners during pregnancy is a fear of harming the baby during sexual activity. As Sabine says, "My only fear at this point is that as my belly grows it could be a real barrier. I can now feel my uterus and am worried that at six to eight months sex will be hurtful to the baby. I probably will be more timid."

In 1999 it was reported that many women avoid intercourse during pregnancy for fear that it may damage the fetus, shorten the pregnancy's duration, or lead to loss of the baby. This same survey of 142 preggies found that most of the women's concerns were not valid, but it also brought to light the fact that only about 30 percent of the women had spoken to their physicians about their sexual concerns during pregnancy, highlighting the need for greater patient-physician communication concerning sex.

Due in part to a lack of supportive reference material, many couples have ill-founded fears and find themselves discouraged from having sex at all. The following are some common fears about sex and pregnancy, accompanied by the realities concerning these fears:

FEAR: Sex during pregnancy will harm the fetus.

REAL DEAL: A 1998 review of fifty-nine studies conducted between 1950 and 1996 on sexual activity during pregnancy concluded that, as long as there are no risk factors (e.g., a sexually transmitted infection), sex *does not* cause harm to the fetus. In fact, a 2001 study, in which 1,853 pregnant women were interviewed, indicated that sexual activity may even have a protective effect against early delivery. Women who reported sexual intercourse both with or without orgasm, and orgasm without intercourse, were likelier to carry their pregnancy to full term than women who didn't engage in sexual activity as late as the twenty-ninth through thirty-sixth week. Furthermore, preterm delivery was significantly reduced among those who engaged in intercourse late in their pregnancy.

FEAR: Sex during pregnancy causes uterine contractions, resulting in premature labor.

REAL DEAL: A study focused on nearly six hundred pregnant women found that women who are sexually active late in pregnancy are *much less likely* to deliver before thirty-seven weeks of gestation than those who are not sexually active. According to their data, orgasmic contractions are *not* harmful to the fetus and will *not* initiate labor.

FEAR: The penis and sperm might harm the fetus.
REAL DEAL: It is physically impossible for the penis and semen to come into contact with the fetus. The uterus is sealed off from the vagina by a mucous plug, which acts as a barrier to ejaculate. And if your partner is worried that his "massive beast" is going to bang up against the baby, you can assure him that your cervix protects your little one from his manliness. "Remember," says Amanda Meulenberg, MD, of New York Downtown Hospital's Department of Obstetrics and Gynecology, "the fetus is surrounded by water and two membranes called the chorion and amnion that provide cushion. Between this protection and the cervix, there is no way the two heads can come into contact."

FEAR: Sex toys are harmful to use during pregnancy.
REAL DEAL: As long as sex toys are cleaned with warm water and soap after every use, and stored in a dry, cool location, sex toys will not harm or invite infection to the mother or her fetus.

FEAR: My preggie may not be up for sex, so I shouldn't bring it up.
REAL DEAL: A preggie may or may not be up for sex, but the only way to find out is to ask her! Many men, like expectant papa Rob, a thirty-one-year-old entrepreneur, admit that they feared imposing any sexual demands on their partner during pregnancy: "I'm really conscious of keeping with my wife's expressed desire. I don't want to be like 'Let's have sex,' because she has a lot going on.

That leads to interesting dynamics, especially since she has masturbated a lot more since getting pregnant."

Our advice to Rob and others: Go ahead and put it out there. Worst-case scenario, she says she's not in the mood and you have to gratify yourself. Chances are, though, that she will take you up on your offer, at least sometimes. Remember the first rule of good communication: The only way to get what you want is to inquire!

While some of the fears we've listed may seem silly or unfounded to you savvier mamas, don't discount the fact that even the least significant of them could play a major role in your lovemaking—or lack thereof. Make sure you and your partner review all of them together and get onto the same page regarding sexual activity during pregnancy. Even the brightest and most well-informed people are susceptible to unfounded fears such as a worry about poking the baby or feeling "watched." Raleigh, a thirty-year-old graduate student and first-time mom-to-be, wrangled with her husband's "three's company" issue very early. "Pirro Cy felt that his daughter was watching," she says. "He had this whole misconception and worry over how sex can harm the child, like can the penis poke the eye out? This, even though ours wasn't a high-risk pregnancy."

🐚 Precautions That Are Justified

While there are many fears and myths about pregnancy that can be countered with scientific fact and research data, there are certain circumstances in which couples should refrain from all sexual intercourse, and others in which a woman should avoid any orgasmic response. *Regardless of whether or not you face one of the following circumstances, you should always consult with a health-care practitioner before deciding that it's okay to have sex during your pregnancy.* According to Dr. Meulenberg, abstinence (defined here as refraining from vaginal-penile, anal, and oral sex, as well as sex acts that can result in climax) is recommended in cases of:

- ❖ placenta previa—a condition where the placenta lies low in the uterus, blocking all or part of the cervix

- ❖ placenta abruption—in which the placenta prematurely separates from the uterine wall

- ❖ multiple fetuses—sex can be safe in early pregnancy, but first check with your health-care provider

- ❖ serious uterine irritability or preterm uterine contractions

- ❖ high risk of premature delivery

- ❖ spotting/bleeding (in some cases)

- ❖ pain

- ❖ past history of miscarriage(s)

- ❖ an incompetent cervix—in which the cervix dilates prematurely and can't "hold in" the fetus

- ❖ an active sexually transmitted infection (yours or your partner's)

- ❖ rupture of the amniotic membranes or leaking of amniotic fluid

As long as you have been cleared by your physician and aren't at risk for any of the above complications, you should be good to go. Lusty thirty-something New Yorker Amanda recalls, "I was at high risk of miscarriage, so I went to a high-risk OB. There was a list of restrictions a mile long about what I shouldn't do, think, say, eat, ride, or wish for. The hardest part for both of us was that once I got a positive pregnancy test, I went on 'total pelvic rest' until the second trimester. That means no penetration, no oral, and absolutely *no orgasms* for ten weeks. My partner, a generous soul, also put himself on hiatus, as a gesture of solidarity. By the time we got to week twelve, it wasn't 'Yea, my baby is alive', it was 'Oh, thank god! We get to have sex again!'"

Always get a second opinion when ordered to abstain, as some physicians have been known to project their own value system onto their patients, including the notion that preggies shouldn't be having sex. Make sure your physician tells you *why* you shouldn't be having sex, then ask for how long and what is meant by "no sex." No intercourse is very different from no sexual contact whatsoever. If you can have orgasms orally or manually (by hand), then we certainly don't want you passing those up! Either way, make sure that you stay informed and empowered as you determine your intimacy potential.

🐾 Sexual Health Considerations

Many couples relish sex during pregnancy for the mere fact that they don't have to worry about birth control. Still, because a number of infections can be spread to your little one during childbirth or in utero, if you or your partner does or may have a sexually transmitted disease, make sure to use protection in the form of a latex condom or, if you're allergic to latex, a polyurethane one. Or just abstain from sex entirely. Here are some thoughts from Dr. Meulenberg, the sassy OB/GYN we introduced you to in our Introduction:

> "Bacterial STDs, like gonorrhea, syphilis, and chlamydia, can lead to severe problems with the fetus, including mental retardation and death. As far as viral STDs go, genital warts are not so worrisome, but herpes can be, especially since condoms are not always protective. Furthermore, if a woman contracts herpes and delivers vaginally during the first outbreak, the fetus can suffer very serious, potentially fatal complications. If a woman has a herpes outbreak when she goes into labor, a cesarean is indicated. Women with a history of multiple outbreaks who want to deliver vaginally can be put on suppressive therapy during their third trimester."

(Note: If you have or may have genital herpes, be sure to tell your doctor or midwife so that plans can be made for the delivery.)

A special caution: Both partners may be at higher risk of contracting HIV from engaging in sex during pregnancy. While part of this increased risk may be due to riskier behaviors—for example, not using a condom—in 2005 researchers concluded that it may also be linked to hormonal changes that affect the genital-tract mucosa or immune responses. If there's a chance you could be at risk for acquiring HIV, and if you choose not to abstain during pregnancy, make sure to use a latex or polyurethane condom.

🐚 The Ride of Your Life

Pregnancy can be an emotional, libidinous sexcapade, or a sensual nosedive, depending in large part on your reaction to the very dramatic changes your body is undergoing, most of which neither sound nor feel very sexy. Your heart is pumping nearly twice the normal volume of blood, your lungs are sucking in more air, and your musculoskeletal system is loaded with a lot more weight. Your digestive system is processing nutrients at an extremely efficient pace, which may be difficult to believe for those experiencing pregnancy's special blend of constipation, heartburn, indigestion, flatulence, and/or nearly incessant urination. All of this, coupled with pregnancy's inevitable exhaustion, may find you choosing the sexual sidelines at times. This is perfectly acceptable; however, we are about to explore some sex-friendly solutions to help keep you booty-licious in the boudoir.

First, let's discuss a few more of pregnancy's physical and emotional changes: The ligaments of your pelvic girdle will stretch enough to allow your uterus to expand up to one thousand times its normal volume. Imagine stretching anything to one thousand times its normal capacity and you'll gain insight as to why you're feeling more than just a little "off." As if that weren't enough, water retention, leg cramps, backaches, and hemorrhoids could cramp your style and deflate your self-image, leaving you feeling less than erotic. Hormonal mayhem may inspire all sorts of mood

How You Can Help Her

While all this growing and blooming can seem beautiful in theory, going through it can be downright awkward, uncomfortable, and terrifying for some women. Your preggie needs increased affection, protection, and love to buffer any feelings of loneliness, isolation, and vulnerability. Besides continuing to express your need and feelings for her, be clear, simple, and nonjudgmental when communicating with her.

—[**for partners**]—

swings. Fortunately, those can include a speedy metamorphosis from tired preggie to saucy tart!

You may find it hard to believe, but those infamous hormonal surges can actually increase your orgasmic potential. Yet they may also leave you feeling a wee bit edgy, moody, exhausted, or even "bipolar"—some of which can be quite sexy, depending on the situation, your partner, and life's other demands. As Allison, a thirty-three-year-old Hot Mama and program coordinator who is expecting her second, explains, "During my first pregnancy, my hormones soared and I wanted my husband all the time. But with my second one—I think part of it is having a toddler—I'm tired and busy. Plus, the hormones of this pregnancy have me in a bad mood, and my husband becomes the object of that anger. I do try to encourage him to be intimate with me, though."

🕏 Embracing Preggie Jekyll/Ms. Hyde

If you're feeling like Dr. Jekyll/Ms. Hyde—longing for more love-making one second, more space the next—you're not alone. You may find yourself surrendering to a mind-numbing fatigue, then raring to go a moment later. Your mood may swing from one that includes grunting, panting, primal lust to one of utter disinterest or disgust at the mere thought of sex. You may find yourself in tears one minute, laughing hysterically the next. Guess what? It's all perfectly normal. Knowing that extreme mood swings are a near certainty can help you and your partner avoid blowups and other love-killers. When the hormonal frenzy gets the best of you, save your love life with a few deep breaths and a little patience.

Your first order of business must be to relax and accept the dramatic changes pregnancy is foisting upon you. Gaining a level of perspective and insight into what's going on with your hormones will not only alleviate some of your emotional reactivity, but can actually turn those raging hormones to your benefit. Pregnancy causes genital engorgement and triggers a surge of love hormones—and we're here to help you acknowledge, celebrate, and take advantage of those facts! Learning to ride the hormonal surges of early pregnancy into multiple orgasms and mind-blowing ecstasy can be one of life's most rewarding experiences.

Remember, you are only pregnant for a short while, so any enhanced sexual potential must be exploited straightaway. Here's more from Sabine, whom we first met earlier in this chapter: "My hormones fluctuate, with the only noticeable change occurring in my skin, causing zits. That's a little embarrassing, but certainly

WHAT'S GOING ON WITH YOUR PARTNER

Remember, in the face of your extreme hormonal responses, your partner may be feeling shut out, confused, and helpless. These fluctuations can have a significant impact on sexual intimacy, especially if your lover's fear of upsetting you puts him or her into a complete avoidance mode. Therefore, it's vital for both of you to practice a lot of patience, forced or natural, and to communicate more than ever. Making a special effort from the get-go to discuss intimacy and to let your lover know how and what you're feeling will keep you connected in terms of wants, needs, and concerns. Getting and keeping things in the open will help you address issues, meet each other's desires, and maintain a sense of shared experience. It took the two of you to get here, so share!

─────────────────[**for hot mamas**]─────────────────

doesn't prevent me from having sex! I think sex is as wonderful and orgasmic, if not better, now that I've gotten over my nausea and fatigue."

The libidinous urgings of early pregnancy can be so great that some women have scared or exhausted their partners with their ravenous sexual appetites. Pregnancy's hormonal cocktail can put your pleasure zones on high alert, which, coupled with the physical changes of early pregnancy, can leave you feeling a bit—ahem— moist at the slightest sexual innuendo. You may even find your clitoral region standing at full attention most of the day, which can be either annoying and distracting or breathtaking and magnificent, depending on your preference and mood.

🖋 Sexy Preggie Tricks of the Trade

Every sexy lady has a few tricks up her sleeve for maximizing her sensuality quotient. Sexy preggies are no different. In fact, they're forced to be craftier than usual. Talk to any Hot Mama about her secret weapons and she's likely to divulge one or more of the tips discussed below.

1. Be the Babelicious Beauty You Are

Think of yourself as a red-hot, modern woman with child. Luscious, ripe, bun-in-the-oven babes with attitude are back in force after being out of vogue for thousands of years. Check magazines and tabloids from the last decade for photos of women like Angelina Jolie, Jada Pinkett Smith, Mariska Hargitay, and Cynthia Nixon to be reminded of how sassy, stylish, and sexy pregnant bodies can be. Who can forget super hottie with tottie Catherine Zeta Jones at the Oscars, getting her sexy on in front of millions of viewers at five and a half months? Talk about inspiration!

Feeling it? Go ahead—in the comfort of your own home, practice your catwalk. Doing it in the nude and in front of a mirror adds an entirely new, breathtaking element to your performance. Do your diva strut wearing heels, a cleavage-enhancing bustier, or whatever floats your Hot Mama boat to get you—and your lover—in the mood. Your lover's positive reaction to your new curves can do wonders to encourage your sensual self to come out and play. As Raleigh recounts, "I walk around the house in my bra and underwear more than I used to, since Pirro Cy loves seeing my body. He's like, 'Look at that belly!' He loves that I'm carrying his child. We're more one now."

So go on—play up your derriere, flaunt your gams, show off your cleavage, and for God's sake invest in a few maternity staples—such as a Hot Mama tank top—to make you feel not just presentable, but pretty. Do it early, confronting head-on any issues that may arise concerning your self-image. It's all about prevention and preparation.

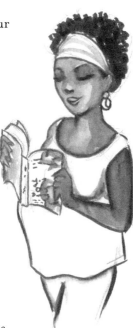

Try casual clothes from the retailers listed in Chapter 5, some of whose products allowed Danielle to outfit herself in Hot Mama fashion for the whole nine months of her spike-heeled pregnancy (when she earned the nickname "Boots"). She was hit on by conservative-looking men who'd have been loath to approach her in a nonpregnant state. By rocking the sexy side of pregnancy attire, Danielle found, to her surprise, that men and women alike were enraptured by a budding belly in tastefully suggestive garb. You are still 100 percent woman, so play it up!

FIGURE 1.1
A preggie in
Hot Mama mode

Have a navel piercing? Although doctors typically recommend having it removed at six months, wearing jewelry with a flexible shaft is an option for those wanting to keep their sexy, rock-star belly rings and studs. Check out www.pregnancypiercings.com.

2. Be Kind to Yourself

Everyone knows that women can be more than a little tough on themselves, especially in terms of their figures. Should you find yourself cursing your form, ask yourself sincerely whether you would ever say anything so harsh to another woman, especially one you cared about and saw every day. Would you be so cruel and critical? Could you? Chances are, you wouldn't dream of it. You would lend some encouragement, a compliment, an uplifting statement. Please, do unto yourself as you would do unto others. Basically, being hypercritical of yourself is the surest way to guarantee that you (and your lover) won't be wanting much sex play, so don't do it! It doesn't do anybody any good.

Feeling "ripe" or "full" is a frequent claim of pregnant women; capitalize on it by imagining your body as ripened fruit begging to be savored, sucked, and enjoyed. Realize that your self-concept is constantly "under the influence" during pregnancy. Hormones can have downright freakish effects on your mojo, so take the upper hand by focusing on your thickening hair, stronger nails, and blood-engorged lips (both sets). Relish the postcoital glow bolstered by increased blood flow to your erogenous zones and also by the nutritive boost you're receiving from your prenatal vitamins. You're experiencing enough estrogen output from your ovaries to fuel a nonpregnant woman for three years (yes, three years), which may at times give you a heightened sense of well-being, tranquility, and contentment. Take advantage of these moments before other hormones kick in and produce different reactions.

3. Remember That You Are What You Eat

Eating wisely when pregnant has nothing to do with obsessing over calories and feeling badly about how you look. Rather, it helps boost your self-esteem by helping you to feel better about yourself and in the skin you're in. Do not buy into the fallacy that pregnancy is a food free-for-all. Your body only requires an additional three hundred calories per day to sustain its pregnant self. It's untrue that all pregnant women polish off an entire bag of Doritos or a pint of Häagen Dazs after dinner—or that they can get away with "eating for two." One survey found that one-quarter of couples (yep, that includes the partner) put on more weight than they should during pregnancy, with a third of women admitting to cravings, especially fruit and orange juice (which aren't bad), as well as pickled foods, bacon, and chocolate (pretty much no-no's, except in very limited amounts).

Thankfully, many Hot Mamas are choosing healthy nibbles and staying trim, and they are becoming more energized in the process. If you're not convinced that eating only an additional three hundred calories or so won't starve your fetus, take a look at medical reviews and reputable online publications, like WebMD.com. Or talk to any mothers you know who belong to the

Baby Boomer generation whose doctors often advised those with "high-risk" pregnancies to consume no more than twelve hundred calories per day to keep the baby's size down—words of "wisdom" volunteered by Danielle's aunt and a group of her friends over brunch at the beginning of Danielle's pregnancy. Obviously, twelve hundred calories is barely enough to sustain even an inactive woman of any age, so this is not exactly sage advice. What we're getting at is the fact that there are a number of less than helpful myths out there about a preggie's diet.

Dr. Meulenberg gives women the following advice about eating during pregnancy:

> Pregnancy is *not* an excuse to overeat. Women who gain too much weight during pregnancy are putting their babies at risk of being too large, a condition which is called fetal macrosomia. When a fetus is too large it can lead to trauma to both the fetus and mother during birth. Trauma to the fetus may include a broken shoulder or nerve damage in the arms, which may resolve or may be permanent. Mothers who have large babies are putting themselves at risk for perineal tears, which can result in fecal incontinence or bladder injury. A large baby will also increase your risk of having a cesarean section because the head may be too large to fit through the pelvis, a condition called cephalopelvic disproportion.
>
> Not eating enough can also be problematic, leading to growth retardation of the fetus. Women need at least seventeen hundred calories per day when pregnant. Once she's in

the second trimester, a pregnant woman should be gaining one to two pounds per week, and twenty to thirty pounds total. At each prenatal visit mothers should be weighed and the size of their uterus measured. If they are gaining too much or too little, or if the uterus is not growing appropriately, action should be taken by the health-care provider.

You see, even your diet during pregnancy affects both your sex life and your baby. Perineal tears make it harder to resume sexual activity postbirth. In an effort to protect both you and your baby, stick with wholesome, healthy foods, which will keep your blood sugar stable, your energy levels up, and your size down.

If you do go a bit overboard and end up giving into one of those craving-induced, animal-like binges, know that sexual activity will help burn some of the extra calories you've consumed. Medical research shows that fifteen minutes of intense foreplay burns over twenty-two calories, depending on your body composition; intercourse of the same duration melts somewhere around sixty-eight calories. Combine these two sexual activities to work off that mini-sundae, handful of Cheetos, or bagful of Pirate's Booty you just scarfed down. And don't forget to let your sweetie know how helpful he or she is being by loving you down to a smaller size!

4. Get Out!

You may find yourself feeling more "whale" than "tail," preferring hibernation to sexing or socializing. Some women find that the no-wine, no-cocktail rule makes it both tougher to loosen up in the bedroom and downright depressing to venture out on the town. Although steering clear of alcohol, cigarettes, and other potentially harmful substances is important, Hot Mamas know that staying connected to their social-support network is equally critical. No Hot Mama stays under self-imposed house arrest simply because of the toxic temptations indigenous to her social scene. So get out, no excuses!

Hot Mamas are not couch potatoes—unless, of course, they're keeping the home fires burning with some stimulating sex play on said sofa. If you're not busy getting "bootay," get your booty off the sofa and out the door! Dress in a flattering ensemble, do your hair and makeup, and boost your positive attitude by maintaining a sense of normalcy.

By continuing to do most of the activities you did before you were pregnant, you will not only send the message that you are a Hot Mama taking charge of her pregnancy, but you will gain confidence in your ability to handle your pregnant body. Letting your hair down and relaxing with your partner or friends can only make for better bedroom time, especially once you've had person after person admire the midriff you're bearing in your sexy getup. Most women who get out often will tell you that they are friskier and more energetic, both in and out of the sack.

When you're out, however, be aware that you may encounter societal notions concerning the "shoulds" and "should nots" of pregnancy. Don't let other people's ideas prevent you from enjoying quality time with your inner circle. Raleigh knows this peril well. "My friends took me out for my birthday, and I ordered a nonalcoholic beer. The waiter poured my drink and regretfully took the bottle immediately, leaving people to critically stare at me for the rest of my meal because they thought I was getting soused. People's judgment is one of the reasons why I don't go out that much. A guy came up to me and said, 'I didn't know they let pregnant women in bars,' like I'm supposed to be home knitting or something. My husband was really upset about it."

We are, too! Nobody should say something so insulting! All we can suggest is to grow a thick skin. But you already knew to do that, didn't you, Hot Mama?

5. Give It an E for Effort

While we consider ourselves your biggest cheerleaders for maintaining quality time in the boudoir during your pregnancy, we don't want to downplay the fact that mommies-to-be and their lovers don't always feel particularly amorous. In fact, like all good things, keeping your love life smokin' takes concentration and effort. But no worries. This is the good kind of work. The payoff is huge.

In order to keep your sex life alive during pregnancy, there simply must be a conscious effort and commitment to do so on the part of both partners. At the very least, pledge to keep things between you warm and comforting. This is a perfect and crucial time to become closer than ever as friends and lovers. Revive your crush on each other. Set aside time every day or week to hold, fondle, and celebrate one other. Indulge your urge to place your hands all over that beautiful belly. As unromantic as it may sound

HOW YOU CAN HELP HER

Many partners are wonderful about showing support for their preggies by abstaining from alcohol and other recreational substances during her nine-month "sentence." Your participation in her lifestyle restrictions makes it easier for her to refrain from those indulgences, and, once again, makes this a team effort. Furthermore, many friends are willing to help the cause by ordering virgin drinks when the group is out on the town. Most good friends would prefer spending time in the company of their pregnant pal to getting drunk, so we encourage you to drum up support from the troops, which will help your Hot Mama to feel loved and supported.

for partners

to some, scheduling time for intimacy, to make sure that it happens regularly, is the cornerstone of many fabulously erotic partnerships. Cuddle, touch, kiss, lick, hug, massage, fondle, and taste each other, even if only for five minutes a day. Felicity says, "My partner loved every second of my pregnancy and our intimacy. He was very loving, making it a wonderful experience."

Hot Mama, are you remembering to be loving to your partner? Sex and intimacy are a two-way street, friend. Don't forget that this can be a delicate time for your significant other.

6. Stay Flexible

Flexibility is key to maintaining an active sex life throughout your pregnancy—and we're not talking about Cirque du Soleil–style contortionism. Staying open-minded about different types of sex play is essential to remaining connected with your partner and having a brilliant time of it. As you navigate your options, be aware that there is no one "right way" to have sex during pregnancy. Everything depends solely on your and your partner's preferences and comfort levels. Many couples find that their preferences don't change much during pregnancy, but others find that they experience all things sexual in a completely altered way. You may find yourself needing less foreplay, for example, given the enhanced blood flow to your genitals.

The important thing is that the two of you do not limit your imaginations. As your body changes, so will your range of options, causing you to exclude some activities and add others. Keeping things fresh, revisiting forgotten sensual pleasures, and having an adventurous mindset will make your quest wildly, erotically successful. The most important thing—and we cannot emphasize this enough—is to surrender yourself every step of the way. Submerge yourself in the most incredible experience of your life. You never know what it may hold for you and your lover.

7. Spoil Yourself

Even if you've never truly pampered yourself, start now. Danielle will attest that regularly napping, going for bikini waxes, and getting facials made a huge difference in her mood and stress level, especially when coupled with staying in shape and focusing on good nutrition. If you've never been crazy about these sorts of self-indulgences, you will be shocked by their feel-good effects. Treating yourself like a goddess translates into feeling like a queen (which may inspire your partner to spoil you accordingly). Felicity feels that maintaining a pampering routine was good for her relationship and her sense of self-worth and confidence, both of which are vital to sexual desire. "I still got waxed and pedicures," she says, "plus went for maternal massages and fitness classes. I tried to stay in shape and definitely ate well. I got my hair cut and did things like that to make me feel groomed and put together. It's important to use tools that help you feel polished." (See Chapter 5 for an inspiring list of ways to pamper yourself over the next nine months.)

8. Know That Your Experience Is Unique

Never compare yourself to other preggies! This no-win game will only leave you feeling insecure. Rather, focus on the love you have, your wonderfully fertile body, the heightened sensations you're capable of experiencing now, and the pleasure of discovering unexplored territory with your partner and yourself.

For Hot Mama Felicity, mother of two boys, sex during her first pregnancy was much more powerful during the first trimester: "Lovemaking was special and more intense at the beginning, knowing that I was sustaining a life. This translated into our intimacy." Her second pregnancy, however, was beset by endless nausea. "I gained only fifteen pounds total, having lost weight during my first trimester because I was so nauseous. While I'd felt attractive and sexy during my first pregnancy, with my second, I was more concerned about the baby growing enough. My attention was on nourishing myself properly more than anything."

Bottom line: Don't size up your licentious sex drive and strong need for loving—or your lack thereof—as "normal" or "abnormal" based on what your mom, sister, best friend, research, or even this book tells you. A wide variety of experiences relating to your sex life throughout pregnancy and postbirth can be regarded as perfectly normal.

❦ Watching the Delivery: How It May Impact Your Sex Life

Here's something to begin thinking about early in your pregnancy. Having your partner in the delivery room could have a significant and positive impact on your relationship as you share one of life's priceless moments. Yet viewing things from the "tail end" of the action, so to speak, may alter a man's perception of sex as he watches his play zone getting ripped and stretched. A handful of studies on a partner's presence at the birth yield mixed results concerning its effect on coital activity or sexual enjoyment for either partner after the fact. The large majority of the partners at Dr. Meulenberg's hospital do not watch. "I personally do not recommend it," she says. "Birth is beautiful, but can be pretty shocking the first time you see it. Lots of partners will get very lightheaded and even pass out when they see the large amount of blood involved. If the partner faints, the moment can be ruined.

I have the partners go to the head of the bed and hold the mother's hand during the final stages of pushing. I feel that it is more important for them to provide emotional support and encouragement."

Here are Danielle's thoughts on the matter:

In my case, my partner saw plenty of vaginal-expulsion action during childbirth class, which I consider vital for *any* partner to watch. Then he opted out of seeing me from that angle on our big day. I am completely grateful for that, because I know him intimately enough to realize that the image would be tough for him to banish from his mind. Had he been a different sort—for example, a doctor—things might have been different. This is a very intimate, delicate, and personal decision, and it should be approached without judgment. You should not insist that your partner view the birth from a position between your legs when he can be every bit as valuable and supportive standing next to your head. Furthermore, his standing at the head of the bed allows both of you to see things from the same angle and to have the same introduction to your new baby. He doesn't get first dibs! Given all of the hard effort I'd put into getting my babe there, I was happy for that, as well.

A sex-positive pregnancy should not be something that only a few lucky women happen upon by chance. Rather, every pregnant woman should feel empowered to enjoy satisfying and fulfilling

HOW YOU CAN HELP HER

There will be times when your preggie truly has no conscious awareness of what she does. You may have to swallow your pride and humor her in some extremely bizarre ways. Consider it in your best interest to keep the peace if you wish to have any hope of intimacy once her hormones get back under control. Here's Raleigh: "During the first trimester, there was a time when Pirro Cy's breath smelled like urine to me. But everything else did, too. So I was always giving him breath mints."

[for partners]

sex. Provided that you're willing to embrace the vast pleasure potential your body will offer for the next nine months, you may never experience more or better sex. So buckle up, Hot Mama-in-the-making. We're about to explore how you can reach the most thrillingly orgasmic, full-body sexual peaks of your life!

2

First Trimester Sex: Can't Get Enough or Can't Get Any?

"One of the greatest sexual benefits of pregnancy is the increased intensity and pleasure of orgasm that usually accompanies sex during pregnancy."

*P*regnancy may have a significant, life-changing impact on your sexuality, or virtually none at all. Most women experience changes in desire for, satisfaction with, and frequency of sexual activity as pregnancy progresses. Some experience this transformation almost immediately after becoming pregnant; others go months with little or no effect.

If you're not on doctor's orders to abstain but are considering sexual activity, take note that many women express regret at having not been sexually active during pregnancy, especially given the time it takes postbirth to get back on track in the sack. Research has found that relationship satisfaction tends to increase slightly during pregnancy, when many couples become emotionally closer as they eagerly anticipate their new arrival. Mutual happiness, however, tends to decrease greatly *after* the birth of a couple's first child, with sexual intimacy being the most vulnerable area, according to a 1998 meta-analysis of fifty-nine studies.

Research has also found that 58 percent of the pregnant women studied experienced decreased sexual desire during pregnancy, while 42 percent reported that theirs stayed the same or increased. By contrast, it has been reported that 82 percent of women think that pregnant women who are able to should engage in intercourse throughout their entire pregnancies in an effort to stay connected to themselves and their partners.

What about same-sex couples? A 1999 study of expectant lesbian couples found that over 85 percent reported greater closeness during pregnancy. Over 53 percent reported improved communication. Almost 83 percent reported less frequent sex, but since more than 87 percent claimed greater relationship satisfaction overall, who are we to say that's necessarily a bad thing?

So if you need greater incentive to keep the home fires burning during pregnancy, find it in the fact that maintaining intimacy during those nine months will help you and your partner make the transition more easily into the all-important period immediately following the birth. Once the new baby arrives, engaging in intimate, caring, and—yes—sexual touch will enhance your connection until you're able to reintroduce your full range of sexual activities.

☞ Sexual Desire During Your First Trimester

You may find yourself all over the map when it comes to sexual appetite during your first trimester (T1), some days feeling ravenous and others disinterested. Or you may sail through this stage as your same ol' sexual self. Most women report that their sexual interest and activity during T1, defined as the time from your last menstrual period to the twelfth week of gestation, either remains unchanged or decreases slightly. Among the culprits that can dampen desire are physical and emotional changes, morning sickness, and fatigue. Extra blood to the genitals may result in discomfort, irritation, and abrasion, depending on your tolerance and sensitivity level. Add to these side effects the initial shock and awe of pregnancy, which can leave some women feeling out of sorts, and you may find your sex life nonexistent.

The good news for women whose sex drives plummet in the beginning of pregnancy is that libido usually rebounds very early in the second trimester (T2). Many women enjoy the first orgasms of their lives or their first multiple orgasms during T2.

Nausea may be a major factor in sidelining your sex drive during T1. For those of you whose "morning" sickness turns into an all-day, every day affair, fear not. This difficulty frequently gives way to a rather easy second trimester. Indeed, some of the women we interviewed who endured the most extreme cases of pregnancy-related nausea turned into some of the sassier, randier Hot Mamas during middle pregnancy. Perhaps it can be chalked up to an utter appreciation for feeling good again. Whatever it is, know that you *will* get to enjoy your blossoming body before long. Still, despite the nausea, you may feel like you're walking on air, elated with the news of your pregnancy. And nothing can make a gal feel sexier in quite the same way!

At the opposite end of the spectrum, some lucky ladies experience increased sexual urges during T1 that often continue or increase through T2. Many of these preggies report an increase in sexual activity, awareness, and interest, often at levels exceeding their normal state. This has been the case for Raleigh: "I noticed major changes from the time I knew I was pregnant. There was a definite increase in my libido and it has stayed more elevated than my norm throughout."

In most cases this heightened sexual desire is due to the sharp spike in estrogen triggered by the onset of pregnancy. The resulting increase in vaginal lubrication and the engorgement of your genitals (known as vasocongestion), with or without sexual arousal, coupled with increased overall vulval sensitivity, can amp

---

WHAT'S GOING ON WITH YOUR PARTNER

Your lover may be feeling his or her own set of pregnancy-related emotions, perhaps becoming more prim and proper than animalistic in response to your newfound sexy surge, especially if he or she takes issue with the notion of sexy preggies. Your partner may begin to feel a bit "used" because of the demand to satisfy your bursts of horniness, especially if your hormonal rush has you swinging from raging anger to pleas for frenzied makeup sex within a five-minute span. Let your partner know it's nothing personal—you're just craving sex in ways you've never known, and it's equally confusing for you.

—[**for hot mamas**]—

---

up your titillation quotient and your desire. Your entire lower body may be constantly awash in pleasurable sensations. Orgasms may come more easily than you could have ever imagined. Lubrication and orgasm may intensify dramatically as the abdominal wall stretches and grows tauter around your lower abdomen, causing the skin that connects your vulva to your lower abdominal muscles to stretch tighter and tighter. Even without any manual stimulation, you may feel your genital area rubbing across the underlying muscles, providing sensations much like those bestowed by any skilled "cunning linguist."

For women who enjoy good clitoral stimulation (and who doesn't, for god's sake), this may be one of the horniest times of your life. Wearing undergarments will only add to the torture. Talk about one Hot 'n' Bothered Mama! For me (Danielle), the skirt-no-panties thing was rough in the winter, especially in the northeastern United States, where I live, but I was forced on several occasions to brave the cold, even in the face of the threat of popsicle privates and all. Vive la crotchless underwear and long, button-to-the-floor winter coats! Many a pair of sweater tights lost its crotch as winter turned bitter and my clit seemed to take on a mind of its own.

℘ Blush-Inducing Dreams

Yet another delicious side effect of being pregnant is a marked increase in sizzling sex dreams. A 1980 study found that 17 percent of those surveyed felt they had many more erotic dreams during pregnancy than usual. In part, this is because a preggie's REM sleep patterns change, leading to more dreams; in addition, her sleep tends to be lighter, making for better dream recall. Danielle's dreams were extremely vivid and very physical, frequently resulting in nocturnal climax.

Based on our discussions with pregnant women nationwide, it turns out that this phenomenon is surprisingly common. Many Hot Mamas confessed that their erotic dreams featured members of both sexes, parties with people other than their partners, multiple partners, typically "unspeakable" sex acts (often shocking to even the hottest Hot Mama), and "strange" and "unusual" sexual activities. One woman claimed to have dreamt of sleeping with nearly every man she'd ever been involved with, except her current partner. Raleigh is still surprised by her pregnancy dreams, which involve everything from girl-on-girl action, orgies, and penetration to feeling sensations against the side of her vagina (as well as a few unmentionables). "The weird thing has been the erotic nature of my dreams and the heightened level of fantasy, because it's totally not something that would turn me on normally," she says. "I've talked to Pirro Cy about it, but none are anything we would want to act on. It doesn't turn me on outside the fantasy element. In fact, it makes me nauseous thinking about some of it. Most of it is me being a voyeur and watching it being done. I totally wasn't expecting these dreams."

Our recommendation: Embrace the dreams. They can offer amazing release—and they can provide great fantasy material for solo or partnered sexcapades when you're awake. Allison says, "My sexual fantasies definitely increased during my first pregnancy. I think it's because I was carrying a boy and had more testosterone—maybe? Anyway, it boosted activity with my husband, which was even more enjoyable since my orgasms involved my entire uterus (and felt like a huge cramp), which was more gratifying."

Here are some pointers for how to remember your sex dreams. Dream experts recommend staying very still in the first moments after you wake, keeping any memories from the dream fresh for your conscious mind to grasp. Write your recollections immediately in a bedside dream journal—one of the most effective training tools for dream recall. Keep track of any additional images that return to you throughout the day to create your own private *Penthouse Forum*-style fantasy collection to pore over with your partner.

Sharing the erotic details of your dreams with your partner can act as a reminder that you are still a sexual being. Your lover is likely to get totally turned on by hearing your stories. He or she will appreciate your new, wilder imagination. Who knows—you may work up to some fantasy play, acting out scenarios now or saving them to sex things up postpregnancy, and you may open a whole new door to a broader sex life within the comfortable confines of your relationship. As any Hot Mama knows, sharing fantasies and dreams with your partner can be a powerful, sexual impetus at all times, not just during pregnancy. Plus it can get you more action.

🐝 Sexual Pleasuring During T1

Most women hardly show during the first trimester of their pregnancy, which makes the "hows" of having sex a relative no-brainer. Even without the telltale bump, many women feel riper, fuller, and more carnal than ever during T1, yet some women fail to realize they're pregnant. For those who are aware of their new status, sex play can become a little more cautious or tentative. Positions that put pressure on the abdomen or pound on the clitoris may unnerve some couples, especially if they've suffered prior miscarriages, as thirty-one-year-old Colin, a papa-to-be from the South, can attest: "When it comes to sex, there's definitely a fear, especially in the first trimester. Lori was really tired, and sex wasn't high on the agenda. We'd also had a miscarriage the first time around, which makes me wary in bed, wondering if sex was an element in the miscarriage or not."

While caution is understandable—and in some cases advised—most couples can continue with their normal prepregnancy sex lives, as long as "normal" doesn't include death-defying gymnastics, rough or violent play, or the insertion of oversized objects. This in no way suggests that pregnant sex can't have its wild side. As Jay, whose wife is pregnant with their second child, says, "There's something about my wife being pregnant that changes my outlook on having sex. The whole idea of it is different. You get so used to worrying about getting pregnant and the ramifications of that happening, that when she *is* pregnant, there's a different attitude, making it more fun and relaxed. She's already pregnant, so there's less at stake. That distracting worry is no longer there; nothing can possibly change how things are. There's a possibility of things sizzling even more because sex isn't so high stakes—we can let go a little more."

🍂 Pregnant Sex Equals Better Sex: Your Most Amazing Orgasm Ever

One of the greatest sexual benefits of pregnancy, and one of the main factors motivating us to put out this book, is the increased intensity and pleasure of orgasm that usually accompanies sex during pregnancy. This is due to the increased blood flow to the genitals that comes with pregnancy. If climaxing during sex has been difficult for you, you may finally find your orgasm—or several! In the genitally engorged state of pregnancy, low-friction, often high-labor acts like cunnilingus and missionary position can cause climax with relative ease.

No matter what your orgasmic quotient has been to date, exploit this phase of your life by exploring all roads to the "Big O":

Spontaneous orgasms—Known also as an "extragenital" orgasm, this kind of climax occurs when a woman's erotic thoughts set her off, without any genital contact. In some cases, a spontaneous orgasm may be triggered by having any part of her body touched while she's lost in sexual fantasy or while she's simply going about her daily activities. Whether or not her efforts are intentional, some women can experience orgasm from imagery alone, a phenomenon more popularly referred to as "thinking off." A woman literally thinks her way to orgasm with all of the "naughty" stuff going on her head!

Given the dreams and fantasies bombarding the average preggie, becoming a whiz at spontaneous "O" can be a breeze. And since pregnancy tends to be an intensely spiritual and emotional time, "thinking off" can become a deeper, more pervasive experience for most preggies.

In 1992 ten women ages thirty-two to sixty-seven were examined to determine whether subjective claims of imagery-induced orgasm were accompanied by the same "physiological and perceptual events" usually included in genitally stimulated climax. The results of the study indicated that these women experienced significant increases in heart rate, systolic blood pressure, pupil diameter, and pain detection and tolerance thresholds, whether using self-induced imagery or genital self-stimulation. Adding to the overwhelming physical evidence surrounding women's ability to think themselves to climax, later publications in this area of research also delve into the spiritual and emotional dimensions of spontaneous orgasm.

Nocturnal orgasm—We typically equate nocturnal orgasm with "wet dreams," or a male's sleep-cycle climax. Research conducted in 1983 found that a woman's vaginal responses to vascular engorgement (the female version of penile erections) during REM (rapid-eye-movement) sleep actually occurred with a frequency equal to nocturnal penile erections in men. Furthermore, during non-REM sleep, a woman's vaginal responses occurred more frequently than male penile erections. Everyone dreams about sex at one point or another as they get their nightly zzzzz's, whether they're consciously aware of it or not. For many women, pregnant or otherwise, these dreams end pleasantly with nocturnal orgasm(s). The brain has become so turned on that it forces the body to experience the entire sexual response cycle.

The prospect of nocturnal orgasm for preggies is amplified by those sex dreams and fantasies mentioned earlier. Increase your chances of remembering your nocturnal climax if and when it does happen by practicing the following rituals: (1) think sexy thoughts before you go to bed by inviting scenarios that you may remember the next morning; (2) pursue lucid dreams as you're dozing off, waking up, or partially awake during the lighter parts of your sleep cycle. Most people are capable of lucid dreaming, which simply means remaining conscious of what you dream and mentally controlling the action that occurs in the dream. Heavy breathing and other classic physiological changes of wakeful orgasm may not always take place during lucid dreaming, but your body will definitely feel warmer, calmer, and more rested afterward. You should be left feeling as though you've just awoken from a nice, long nap. And what Hot Mama couldn't use that?

Simultaneous orgasm—For many couples, simultaneous orgasm—when both lovers climax at the same time—is one of lovemaking's highest goals. Yet a coordinated reaction is often elusive for heterosexual couples since many men sail through the sexual response cycle much faster than women. Typically, experts recommend that the man slow down his thrusting sufficiently to allow his partner's sexual response cycle to catch up. During pregnancy, however, you may find that your hypersensitive and sexually charged body not only keeps up with but surpasses your partner's in the speed of its response. Regardless of whether you climax in tandem or separately, always remember that seeing your lover lost in climactic ecstasy, brought on by you, can be the ultimate pleasure.

For same-sex partners, even those usually in synch, achieving simultaneous O can be challenging during pregnancy for the simple reason that the pregnant partner may race to climax well in advance of her partner. Introducing toys and other hyperstimulating accessories for the nonpreggo partner may help her to keep pace. So break out that vibrator and coax yourselves to mutual climax!

Although we have been praising the wonders of engorged genitals, it's only fair to point out a potential drawback. Your genitals may become so sensitive that even the slightest stimulation becomes extremely uncomfortable or downright painful. Most women agree that although getting turned on happens faster during pregnancy, climaxing may take longer because too much of a good thing can be just that—too much. Furthermore, as orgasm approaches, pelvic floor muscles work overtime to clamp down on the urethral area and release waves of climactic pleasure. Lacking sufficient exercise and endurance, these muscles can fatigue, preventing full-blown orgasm.

So what to do? PC muscle exercises. The payoff? More control—and a more intense climax. With improved PC muscle tone your orgasms will be out of this world, a reality your partner should find pretty stimulating as well!

🦢 Meet Your Love Muscle

The following two sections may be the most important in this book. The sooner you can begin exercising your pubococcygeus muscle (PC muscle), the better. A vaginal "strength-training" program not only will help you out on D-day (delivery day), but will also help you get back in the sex saddle sooner after giving birth. Exercising your pubococcygeus muscle—a collective term for the group of pelvic floor muscles that run from pubic bone to tailbone, encircling the base of your vagina, urethra, and rectum—will enhance preggie sex, help you attain orgasm (perhaps even multiple orgasms), and give you stronger and better ones at that. Basically, it puts you in control of your urogenital diaphragm, which in turn benefits your overall sex life.

Commonly known as Kegels, after the doctor who developed and publicized them, these exercises help reduce your chances of vaginal infection by delivering more blood to the vaginal lining. Plus, they help you to grip your partner's finger or penis more strongly during sex, providing your lover with more sensations. A strong PC also makes you feel more sensitive, react more responsively, and feel tighter to your partner. It strengthens vaginal control for delivery of your baby. All these reactions occur in large part because of the pudendal nerve, which runs through the PC muscle and triggers most of its reactions to genital and anal stimulation. This is also the nerve that communicates with your brain to induce the rhythmic contractions associated with most types of orgasm. Lastly, having strong PC muscles boosts your sexual self-confidence. "I really stress Kegels after the onset of pregnancy," says Dr. Meulenberg. "If a woman has had a vaginal delivery she is at increased risk for urinary incontinence and sexual dysfunction after menopause. By starting Kegels early, and keeping those muscles strong throughout pregnancy, women may have fewer problems down the road."

All of the women we spoke to were well aware of the importance of Kegels, having gotten word from their doctors, midwives, and other women. The challenge for practically everyone, however, was remembering to practice them on a regular basis. Here are our recommendations:

- ❖ Record your Kegel exercise regime in your Blackberry or scheduling book.

- ❖ Leave Post-It notes around the house or any place you frequent.

- ❖ Ask your partner to remind you.

- ❖ Start doing Kegel exercises as a part of your daily meditation practice.

Basically, as a reminder to do them, pair your Kegel exercises with anything you do on a regular basis, and you'll be in good (PC) shape.

❧ PC Muscle Exercises: Identifying the Pelvic Floor

The first order of business is to isolate your PC muscle and identify exactly the sensations associated with this area. The easiest way for most women to achieve this is when they're in the bathroom. Try stopping the flow of urine midstream. By contracting your pelvic floor muscles to stop the flow, you are replicating the contractions necessary for vaginal manipulation. In short, you are exercising the PC muscle you want to target. The urethra fastens down in response to vaginal contractions, preventing urine from flowing out. The feeling of clamping down midstream will give you a good sense of which muscles you need to focus on for maximum vaginal tone.

Another option is to push down as though you are having a bowel movement. Do this for several repetitions. During this move, sometimes called "blossoming," you forcefully push your vagina outward, as though you want to express the inside toward the outside to show your partner or display in a mirror for examination. Then, suck your PC muscle back up and in with a contraction, using only the pelvic muscles, located between your legs, to do so. Take care to avoid contracting your abdominal, thigh, or buttocks muscles while performing the exercises. Maintain a neutral spine and visualize "sucking" a penis, finger, or another phallic object into the vaginal cavity using the force of your muscles alone.

FIGURE 2.1
The PC muscles

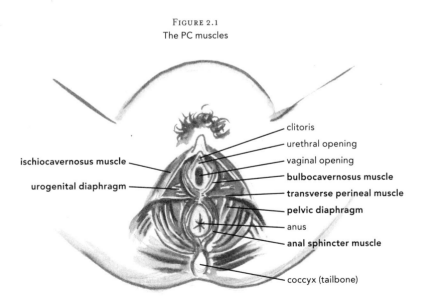

Yet another way to identify the correct muscle group, and one of our favorites, is to insert your finger into the vagina. (If this isn't your cup of tea, a vibrator, dildo, or partner's finger or penis will do.) Once the finger is inside about an inch or so, tighten the muscles of your vulva, as if holding back urine. Notice how the muscles of the vagina squeeze your finger. (If you don't feel the contraction, don't worry. You will after a couple of weeks of exercising your PC.) You may discover that what you thought was a vaginal contraction was more anal-focused or abdomen-focused, in which case you need to adjust your contractions to effect a vaginal squeeze. Varying the tempo and pressure of the contractions around your finger is one of the most effective ways to identify exactly how the muscles in this region work, and doing this offers a wonderful means of varying the movements to utilize the fullest range of motion for the best workout. Plus, the added resistance of the inserted object will help improve your squeezing skills. Your goal is to strengthen this region in preparation for giving birth and to help you "snap back" rapidly afterward.

Once you're comfortable with your ability to locate and contract your PC muscles, it's time to begin a regular routine of toning and training. Below, you'll find a beginner's regimen uniquely geared to achieving maximum results in a minimum amount of time. Prior to engaging in these exercises, breathe deeply into your lower abdomen, filling your side and back lungs. Feel the air filling your lungs all the way up to your throat; then exhale fully to discharge any tension in your midsection. Remember, focus the contractions only on your PC muscles.

> ### How You Can Help Her
>
> *Be her Kegel coach. Remind her to train. Even with the best intentions, a woman's biggest challenge is often simply remembering to do her PC exercises. Sending her a thrice-daily text message or e-mail is a great way to make sure she gets and stays committed to the practice. If she becomes defensive, gently remind her that faithfully doing her exercises will help make D-day easier and faster—and will also make postbirth sex more enjoyable. She can't really argue with that.*
>
> —[**for partners**]—

The beauty of these exercises is that you can do them anywhere —in the subway, at the office, at the dinner table. Usually, though, women find that doing their PC exercises in public is more comfortable once they've had quite a bit of practice. So find a private, quiet space, and let's begin with the most basic PC exercise:

1. Make sure that your bladder is empty.

2. Relax and concentrate on your vagina; focus on contracting only the pelvic floor muscles.

3. Tighten the pelvic floor muscles and hold for three slow counts.

4. Breathe slowly and deeply.

5. Completely relax the PC muscle for three counts.

6. Perform nine contractions, at three counts each, three times a day. Slowly work up to three daily sets of thirty-six contractions.

If you cannot contract your PC muscle for three counts, try holding it for one or two counts while building your strength and endurance. Gradually work up to ten counts per hold.

A word of caution: Take care not to increase the number or frequency of repetitions too quickly, as this will not improve results but rather may cause extreme muscle fatigue and increase the potential for urine leakage. Definitely not sexy!

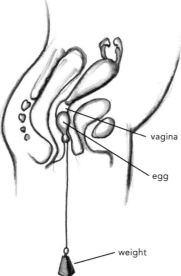

vagina

egg

weight

FIGURE 2.2
Women can use a weight when they practice PC muscle exercises

Next, let's try a more advanced technique, known as the "elevator":

1. Contract the PC muscles as you count to ten, tightening and lifting them as you count.

2. Visualize your vaginal area retreating in and up toward your uterus, as though any object near the opening would be forcibly drawn into the vagina and squeezed tightly.

3. Hold for a count of ten at the peak, the point at which you're sure you cannot draw up or tighten your PC muscles any further.

4. Release slowly as you count to ten, until you bottom out as though your vagina were now expelling the object you earlier pictured drawing in.

What's happening with your breath? Make sure you're not holding it, but rather slowly breathing in and out with your repetitions. Breathing rhythmically also enhances lovemaking. You can squeeze your partner to increase the pleasure for both of you, enabling you to experience a more intense, total-body orgasmic response.

Note that you're doing Kegel exercises *incorrectly* if you experience discomfort in your abdomen or back while performing them. If that happens, stop immediately.

We promise that you will feel motivated to keep up with your Kegel routine once you've experienced the increased skill and desire that goes along with improved PC muscle tone. Who wouldn't want a stronger and better-toned vagina?

Second Trimester Sex: Prepare to Be Tantalized!

"Your breasts are heaving. Your genitals are throbbing. Your whole being is aching. You're literally dripping with anticipation."

"*M*y tiny bump has my partner so excited," says Sabine. "You should see how he talks to it. It's so sweet and sexy." At four months pregnant, Sabine feels sexier than ever. "During sex," she says, "he'll check in with the baby. We refer to the whole sexual experience as 'family bonding.'" This from a woman whose most notable experiences during her first trimester were fatigue and nausea. If that describes you, take heart—there *is* hope!

The "comeback" potential of the second trimester includes a resurgence in energy levels coupled with a sense of joy and wonder as you feel physical stirrings from the babe and witness the first real evidence of her or his existence popping out in front of you. Those of you who enjoyed a no-show first trimester will have to 'fess up now, because there will be no hiding the fact that your "dirty dealings" have you up the duff! For some women, getting past the morning sickness can rekindle the urge to get busy in bed, but an equal number get the heebie-jeebies at the thought of having sex with the child so obviously present. Usually, the pregnant partner is the first to get creeped out at the thought of preggie sex, given the close proximity in which she and the child are living.

If this is the case for you, sit down and have a frank discussion with your honey about any and all sex-while-pregnant hang-ups. Do this to nip the awkward thoughts and feelings in the bud, and also to explore what both of you are comfortable (physically *and* psychologically) doing. Remind yourselves that you're doing this for your baby—that it's in everyone's best interest for you to remain sexually active. As you have this discussion, remember that it is especially important to own your thoughts and feelings with "I" statements. Start sentences with "I feel" or "I think." We point this out because, rather than representing your own true beliefs, much discomfort around this issue may actually stem from societal or religious messages that have been dictated to you—and that don't exactly support intimacy during pregnancy. Using "I" statements will also make your conversation a much more personal and, therefore, valuable one.

🐾 Physical Changes During T2

Before we dive into all of the fun stuff in store for you and your beloved during the second trimester, we need to deal with the elephant in the living room (no, not *you*, silly!). Let's chat a bit about the major changes taking place within your body during this part of your pregnancy. During T2 your body undergoes a complete overhaul. Knowing exactly what's happening will help you stay abreast of things before they catch you off guard.

By the second trimester, defined as the thirteenth through twenty-seventh week of gestation, according to Dr. Meulenberg, you'll likely find yourself either swearing at or reveling in (m)any of the following conditions:

❖ a vagina dripping with moisture (due to higher estrogen levels), at times requiring constant use of panty liners

❖ a swollen (read: *gigantic*) clitoris

❖ labia that throb with increased blood engorgement

❖ emotional highs and lows due to increased levels of estrogen and progesterone, resulting in heightened libido, intensified physiological sensations, and emotional sensitivity

❖ fatigue, absentmindedness, and moodiness due to an increase in progesterone, which has a relaxing effect on your central nervous system

❖ nasal congestion

❖ swelling of the extremities

❖ leg cramps and varicose veins

❖ bloating and gas

❖ hemorrhoids

- ❖ areolas that are deeper in color

- ❖ breasts so big you may need to wear a comfortable bra 24/7

- ❖ extreme nipple sensitivity

- ❖ better skin tone

With all of the physical and emotional upheaval caused by these issues, for better or for worse, you may find yourself rewriting your impression of who you are as a person, as a woman, and as a sexual being, especially when you consider how your sexuality has been rewired in so many ways. Your crown jewel is at its most active, with the potential to deliver more orgasms—and multi-orgasms—than ever. You're wetter, hotter, and lustier, and you're dying for proper sexual attention. As your little one makes itself at home in your belly, you may find yourself examining your new role and trying to define what sort of (Hot Mama) parent you hope to be at both the societal and familial levels.

To top things off, obsessing over your increasing size may cause stress. Many women, even those with a reasonably positive body image, can succumb to the pressures of looking svelte during pregnancy, despite knowing that weight gain is healthy and normal. Add powerful food cravings, which require all your willpower to ward off, and you may find your Hot Mama self a little worse for the wear at times.

Having caved in to a craving once in a while, Danielle knows what it's like to obsess for hours over the calories contained in a few extra Oreos. Still, self-confidence and attitude are everything in

WHAT'S GOING ON WITH YOUR PARTNER

You may not be alone in your physical upheaval. Some men have been known to experience the joys of pregnancy during their part-ner's pregnancy, a phenomenon termed couvade syndrome. Your partner may gain weight, experience nausea, undergo appetite changes (including cravings), and endure mood swings. Basi-cally, he experiences a "sympathetic pregnancy." Up to 90 percent of dads are said to have this experience at some point during the nine months, especially in the last two trimesters. The only cure is birth.

{ **for hot mamas** }

the sex game, whether you're pregnant or not, and you simply have to learn to shut out that mental noise. Arm yourself with an arse-nal of healthy snacks and water to keep your cravings at bay. Blood sugar can drop rapidly during pregnancy, and being prepared for that is a trick you must master. Dr. Meulenberg explains, "Dur-ing pregnancy, the body has an increased resistance to insulin, the hormone that allows you to metabolize sugar. There is also an increased output of insulin during pregnancy. Pregnant women are at risk of developing gestational diabetes"—that is, pregnancy-related diabetes.

Being informed and having a game plan are vital to enjoying every aspect of your pregnancy.

How You Can Help Her

If your preggie is mired in negative attitudes about her changing form, be her personal cheerleader. She can never get enough positive feedback, so tell her how beautiful, incredible, and sexy she is. Encourage sensual activity. Let her know that you want her now more than ever. Don't be afraid to suggest getting sexy, as this can be one of the most effective ways of getting her whipped into proper Hot Mama mental form.

─────────────[**for partners**]─────────────

🐚 Your Body as a Playground

Hot Mama, you have become a veritable sensual playground! For many of you, T2 may be defined more than anything else by the chronic flow of blood to your genitals. A warning about genital engorgement: You'll either love it or loathe it. There is very little middle ground when it comes to the hypersensitive hot zones of pregnancy. Either your fully engorged nipples and clit will bring delightfully on-the-spot orgasmic opportunity, or they will breed such irritation that you'll want to scream. Plenty of women enjoy the all-day clitoral hard-on; others find it maddeningly distracting and annoying. Furthermore, the increased stimulation can cause climax-induced cramping, especially as your growing baby stretches the uterine wall and abdominal muscles.

It's normal for a preggie to experience cramps during and up to a half hour after sex. These cramps may be caused by increased blood flow to the abdomen, prostaglandins in her partner's sperm, or emotional issues. If you are concerned that your cramping may be excessive or abnormal (see box below), be sure to consult a health-care practitioner before making love again.

Throughout Danielle's pregnancy, multiple orgasms would result in sometimes disturbing levels of postcoital cramping. Given her familiarity with the sexual response cycle, these instances were less troublesome than they may have been to someone less knowledgeable. By surrendering to the cramping sensation rather than cringing and fearing it, she was able to achieve a unique pleasure/pain cycle that helped her later in the delivery room.

Learning early to breathe through cramping sensations can be excellent practice for early labor, a time when you need to surrender to the experience of riding the waves of contractions. Your body is taking you on a trip, and being present for the journey without trying to control it can heighten your capacity for pleasure. Remember the law of opposites—pain and pleasure are

---

Postcoital Cramping: When Should You Be Concerned?

According to Dr. Meulenberg, you should seek medical attention "when the pain comes and goes in waves, when the pain doesn't go away within a reasonable time period, when any bleeding is more than just spotting, or when there's a leakage of fluid." She further warns, "Orgasm's release of oxytocin can lead to significant uterine contractions and the onset of labor, especially in the last weeks of pregnancy."

on opposite ends of the same spectrum. They are closely related in the sense that giving in to one can heighten the other. Feeling completely at ease with postorgasmic cramping takes mental conditioning, practice, and a lot of self-talk, but it's worth it. Fortunately, in most cases, these pains are merely irritating rather than debilitating.

Don't get freaked out if your baby gets active during or soon after you've climaxed. A fetus often responds to the uterine contractions of orgasm by kicking and moving about. Danielle's son, Brando, would become quite active as she approached climax, to the point of near-distraction, but it was always worth staying the course. Brando's acrobatics actually made the sensations stronger for Danielle, possibly because her uterus was working overtime to get her to the big O.

❧ Titty-F***ing Mama

Another delight for many women in T2 is an ever-growing voluptuous bosom with deeply rich-colored nipples. For many of you, enhanced breast tissue can add "titty f***ing" to your sexual repertoire for the first time ever. Imagine how pressing your cleavage around your partner's shaft can rekindle the fireworks between you. Bring your partner to arousal with oral or manual stimulation. Stare deeply into his eyes as you use your upper arms to squeeze your breasts tightly together around one very erect member. Incorporate lube to allow enough slippage yet enough friction to bring him either to climax or to the verge. Continue using your hands to stroke, rub, and manipulate as you choose, and watch your partner reach new ecstatic heights. If you can handle it, have your lover tweak your nipples, which are probably more sensitive than ever. This action alone may easily send you into an orgasmic frenzy.

On another breast-related note, you will definitely need a good bra for extra support during this time, so why not select one that's also sexy? Although "erotic" and "supportive" don't always go hand in hand when you're talking about undergarments, you and your partner can make the search a team effort and have fun with it. Pore through all the hysterical, hideous, and heat-inducing possibilities for your "private viewings only" wardrobe. A great place to get started is LSR Maternity (www.lsrmaternity.com). The luxury maternity brand A Pea in the Pod (www.apeainthepod .com) also carries sexy apparel, such as the Elle Macpherson bra line, which offers comfort, style, and pretty lace accents.

For all your maternity clothes, but especially undergarments, always opt for natural, dye-free cottons if you're experiencing any sort of skin irritation. Consider using baby detergents that are free of dyes and fragrances to avoid irritating the hot spot 'tween your thighs.

⚘ Broaden Your Horizons

As you explore and enjoy the vast array of sexperiences available to you and your lover, don't neglect noncoital play. To give you an idea of what others are up to, we've listed some compelling findings an old colleague of Yvonne found on erotic and sexual activities preferred during and after pregnancy:

* nongenital tenderness (preferred by 41–53 percent of lovers surveyed)

* clitoral stimulation (preferred by 25–32 percent)

* breast stimulation (preferred by 23–30 percent)

* vaginal stimulation (preferred by 15–30 percent)

* oral stimulation, man active (preferred by 6–16 percent)

* oral stimulation, woman active (preferred by 4–11 percent)

* anal stimulation (preferred by 0–3 percent)

It's important to keep in mind that some of these numbers are most likely skewed due to social taboos, misinformation about sex during pregnancy, or a lack of know-how regarding safe and doable sexual activities in the presence of a growing belly. Take the statistics with a grain of salt, and approach the material in this chapter with an open mind. Sex during the second trimester and beyond offers you a lot of choices.

The following incentives should also inspire you. Sexual activity helps you:

* Keep weight off—Sex can help burn fat and calories. Some lovers claim benefits like weight loss and increases in strength, flexibility, muscle tone, and cardiovascular conditioning.

* Manage pain—Sex does wonders for lower-back pain in particular.

❖ Combat stress—Sex fights your body's tension by improving your stress response, releasing oxytocin, and stimulating feelings of warmth and relaxation.

❖ Boost intimacy—Sex acts like a relationship glue by sending mood-boosting hormones throughout your and your lover's bodies.

❖ Keep your immune system strong—Sex helps your body ward off ailments.

❖ Sleep better—Sex, including sex with yourself, will help you to sleep more soundly and easily.

❖ Increase your energy and optimism.

❖ Enjoy a shorter labor.

❖ Experience less discomfort during pregnancy and labor.

❖ Decrease fetal stress, resulting in a calmer pregnancy.

⁙ Full-Body Blahs

We haven't forgotten about those of you who aren't enjoying sexual bliss all the time. If you're experiencing the opposite—full-body blahs—don't worry. You're normal. You may simply require more rest, less stress, or a lower-key approach to your sex life while pregnant. Check out the following pointers:

❖ Seek out intimate moments with your partner even when you're not in the mood for sex. Do not allow the blahs to

> #### HOW YOU CAN HELP HER
>
> *Give her loving reassurances that you are there for her and will help her no matter what. Make regular romantic gestures, especially ones involving tender touch. Throughout her pregnancy, her interest in tenderness will stay constant or even increase.*
>
> ─────[**for partners**]─────

interfere with your desire for intimate touch with your partner. In fact, there are few quicker fixes for a really horrible day than a bit of sensual touch or sex play.

❖ Masturbate. Even a small amount of pleasurable self-touch will likely improve your mood and sense of well-being. Masturbation is also known to improve rest and sleep.

❖ Surround yourself with erotic photographs, literature, artwork—whatever turns you on. Even when she's pregnant a woman needs to seduce herself at times.

❖ Tune in to your senses. Everything is enhanced during T2. Food tastes better. Scents are stronger. Music is more intense. Your skin is more receptive. Immerse yourself in this sensory surplus.

Even if some of pregnancy's "side effects" are impacting your game, the more you and your lover are able to be intimate, the better it will be for your body and relationship now and in the long term. It's important to stay connected with regular touch, which is a powerful and important component of closeness during this time. Often underrated, intimate touch is the driving force behind sensuality in late pregnancy. Touch offers physical and emotional benefits such as a boost to your immune system and mood, and the release of oxytocin to enhance sexual arousal, response, and pleasure. Kissing—the long, wet, slow, deep kissing of your presex days—ups the voltage and maintains your connection without requiring the energy of more vigorous sex play.

During any loving touchfest, deciding how far you want to go is entirely up to the two of you, but know that occasionally "taking one for the team" can yield some delightful surprises. You may find yourself feeling caught up in ecstasy when you thought you were ready to roll over and fall asleep. Choose to experience the new sensations and heightened sexual response that are the gifts of pregnancy. Delight yourselves by committing to do the deed as often as you can muster the time and energy. The resulting happiness and good memories will be worth the effort. Jay fondly recalls a postclimactic moment when his wife was carrying their son: "One time, when she had an orgasm, she lay back and said, 'I bet he's going to like that.' And we laughed. We thought that her orgasm had to be a good thing for him—that it would make him feel good."

𝔈 Sexual Positions to Accommodate Your Growing Belly

Your breasts are heaving. Your genitals are throbbing. Your whole being is aching. You're literally dripping with anticipation.

You want sex—no, make that *need* sex—and you want it *now*! Only you're not sure what you should—or are allowed to—do.

During T2 and beyond, it's natural for lovers to find their enthusiasm for eroticism stifled by real and perceived restrictions on what sorts of activities are okay. While positions putting any pressure on a preggie's stomach are absolute no-no's throughout most of your pregnancy (and are probably too uncomfortable anyway), pregnant couples can indulge in a number of basic positions all the way to D-day. These include, but are not limited to, safe variations on: woman-on-top, modified-missionary, side-by-side, rear-entry, standing, and sitting positions.

For these and any other sexual positions you and your partner may engage in during your pregnancy, there are certain rules and cautions that need to be observed:

1. Stick with positions that allow shallow thrusting. Your cervix may be tender or even bleed with deep penetration, especially late in the pregnancy, when it's ripening.

2. Keep your partner's weight *off* your belly and tender breasts. This can be challenging, but it's important.

3. Utilize positions that allow for the woman's control over the depth and angle of penetration (in this way she gets to play cowboy!).

4. Beginning at four months, according to Dr. Joel Evans, coauthor of *The Whole Pregnancy Handbook,* women should not be on their backs for more than five minutes or so.

WHAT'S GOING ON WITH YOUR PARTNER

People have the tendency to see pregnancy as a delicate condition, so remind your lover that you're not fragile—that you can handle business as usual, inside the bed and out. Many people automatically assume that preggies can't take care of themselves, even in everyday activities. Prove that you are autonomous. Danielle worked up to sixty hours a week until just days before she went into labor. Others, including your lover, will admire your feats, which will make you seem even sexier and more desirable. A 1998 study reported that a woman's positive work life was associated with a greater frequency of sexual intercourse during pregnancy, and greater sexual satisfaction and less frequent loss of sexual desire at four months postpartum.

[**for hot mamas**]

5. Avoid positions that require the preggie to twist.

6. Communicate! If you're not jiving with a position, let your lover know. If things need to be switched up, speak up. If you want it harder or faster, take charge.

The following positions offer a wide variety of choices. Use your imagination to make them your own by modifying them. Without further delay, let's have sex!

Note: Although the focus in the following positions is vaginal-penile intercourse (including intercourse with a strap-on dildo), if you're in the mood for anal sex these positions work for that as well.

Woman-on-Top

Especially early in pregnancy, straddling your partner and riding high should pose no challenge at all. Take care to prop yourself upright to avoid exerting undue pressure on the belly. While some pressure on a pregnant woman's belly is often inconsequential, excessive pressure can be fatal to the fetus and should be avoided. Don't lie on your belly or press it too hard against your partner, even in the heat of passion. Doing so can restrict the aorta, stemming the flow of blood to you and your child.

Benefits of Woman-on-Top

~ You receive direct stimulation of the clitoris.

~ Being on top puts you in control of the speed, angle, and depth of vaginal thrusting.

~ You're in charge, which can mean increased pleasure for you if you know what you're doing.

~ Your lover can stimulate your clitoris with his or her fingers.

~ They can play with, touch, and enjoy the sight of your breasts and other parts of your body.

~ Blood will flow more freely to your male partner's erectile tissue, allowing for greater stimulation and pleasure.

~ Being upright can help you avoid nausea.

Start by kissing and embracing as you lie next to each other. Then slowly position yourself so that you're sitting upright on top of your partner, straddling their hips, making sure to put most of your weight on your knees (see Figure 3.1). This position is excellent for late pregnancy.

Lean back on your partner's thighs (see Figure 3.2).

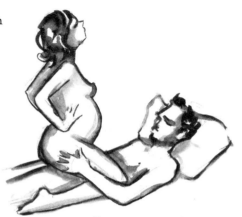

FIGURE 3.1
Woman-on-top position

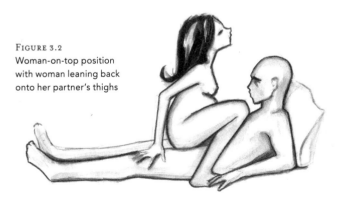

FIGURE 3.2
Woman-on-top position
with woman leaning back
onto her partner's thighs

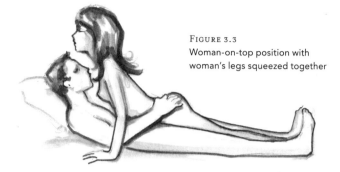

FIGURE 3.3
Woman-on-top position with
woman's legs squeezed together

Variations include:

— To increase friction, squeeze your legs together inside your
partner's to create a snugger genital fit (see Figure 3.3). Use this
position during the first trimester only, as it requires the woman
to place some weight on her belly.

— Turn to face your partner's feet, giving him a full rear view, and
see the sparks fly (see Figure 3.4).

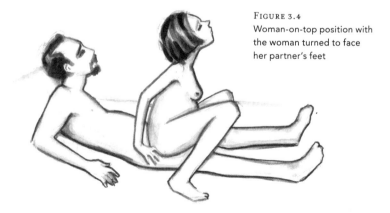

FIGURE 3.4
Woman-on-top position with
the woman turned to face
her partner's feet

HOW YOU CAN HELP HER

It's important to check in with her regularly to learn what feels good and what doesn't —for example, whether she wants her breasts massaged and, if so, how and for how long. Her comfort is of the utmost importance. Also, don't rush. Making her feel cared for, especially as she prepares for her own caretaker role, will increase your shared intimacy. Helping her to relax will enable her to let go in the sack, which will benefit both of you.

{ **for partners** }

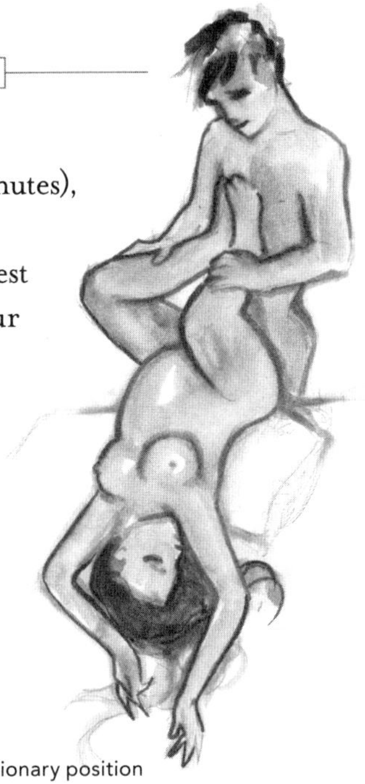

Modified-Missionary (T1 only)

Lie on your back (for no more than five minutes), with your knees open and drawn up toward your chest. Rest your feet on your lover's chest (see Figure 3.5). Putting a pillow under your bum may help. Be sure to communicate as you figure out what is a comfortable, easy thrusting pace.

Benefits of Modified-Missionary

~ Angle allows for clitoral stimulation.

~ It's a relaxed position for you; you don't have to do as much work.

~ You can look into each other's eyes and kiss.

FIGURE 3.5
Modified-missionary position

Other variations include:

— Straightening your legs and resting them against your lover (see Figure 3.6).
— Having your partner kneel between your legs (see Figure 3.7).

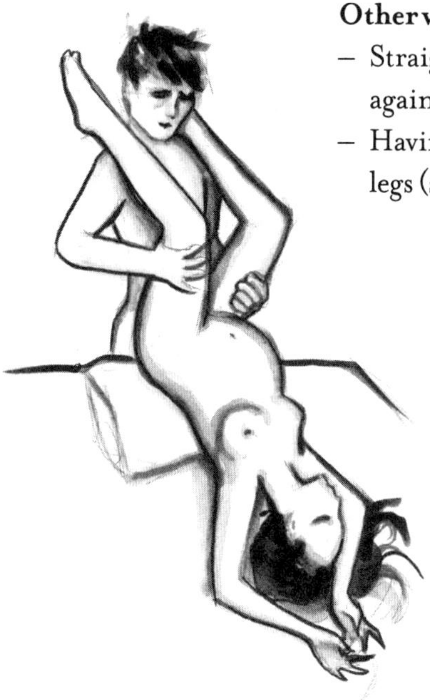

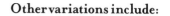

FIGURE 3.6
Modified-missionary
with the woman's legs
straightened out

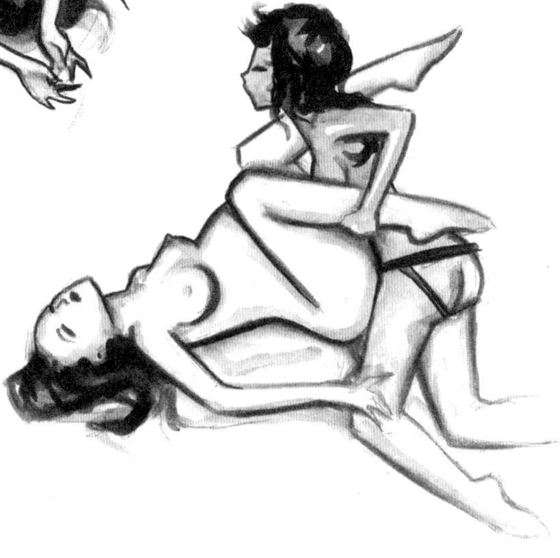

FIGURE 3.7
Modified-missionary
with the preggie's
partner kneeling
between her legs

Lying on your back, with your legs hanging off the side of the bed. Have your partner get down on his or her knees to achieve penetration (see Figure 3.8). A pillow beneath the knees may make this more comfortable.

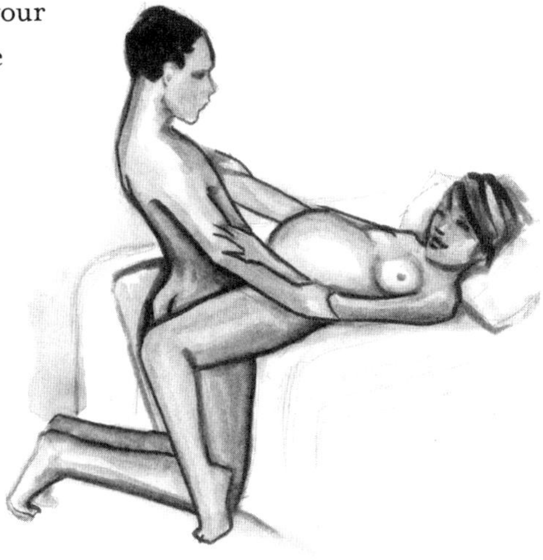

Side-by-Side

Both partners lie on their sides, facing the same way. The pregnant partner draws her legs up to allow easy rear access, affording her partner maximum depth control (see Figure 3.9).

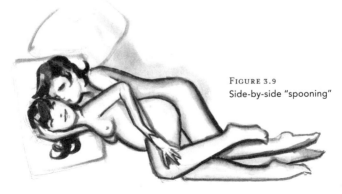

FIGURE 3.8
Modified-missionary with the woman on her back, legs off the side of the bed, and her partner on their knees

FIGURE 3.9
Side-by-side "spooning"

Benefits of Side-by-Side

~ Allows for deep penetration.

~ Your sweetie can stimulate your clitoris as you lean back.

~ Sex can be leisurely, comfortable, relaxing, and can go on for longer than with other positions.

~ Allows for lots of body contact and caressing.

~ You can fall asleep in this cuddle position.

~ The full body contact increases your intimacy.

~ If your lover is well-endowed or using a large dildo, you don't have to deal with as much pressure.

One variation is for partners to lie on their sides, facing each other. Now only you roll back, drawing up your top leg. Your partner can then enter you from the side (see Figure 3.10). Depending upon the position of your lower legs and thighs, differ-

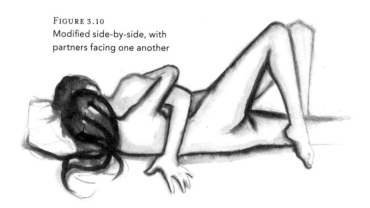

FIGURE 3.10
Modified side-by-side, with
partners facing one another

ent movements are possible and will provide different sensations to your genitals.

Benefits of Modified Side-by-Side

~ Allows for more vulval exposure.

~ The clitoris is more accessible, which allows for easier clitoral stimulation and climax.

~ Ideal in late pregnancy since it allows space for your belly between you and your partner.

~ Your partner's thrusting can be more easily restricted.

Rear-Entry

For the classic "doggie-style" position, get on all fours and have your partner get on their knees so that they can enter you from behind (see Figure 3.11). This will allow for deep thrusting that increases G-spot stimulation, though you will need to make sure that your partner doesn't thrust too deeply.

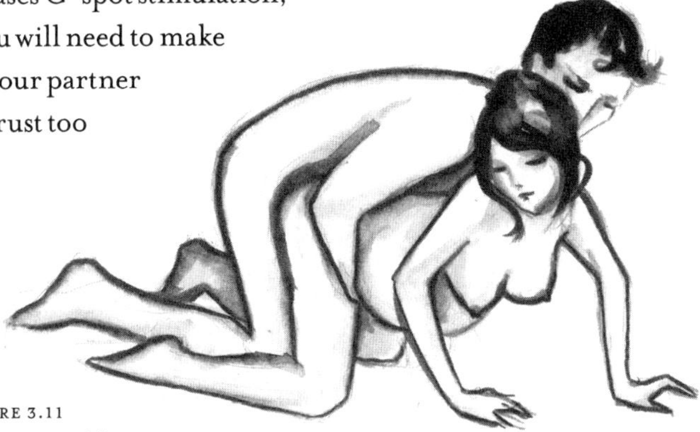

FIGURE 3.11
Rear-entry position

Benefits of Rear-Entry

~ Plenty of room for the belly.

~ Either of you can stimulate the clitoris.

~ Great position if you're experiencing backaches.

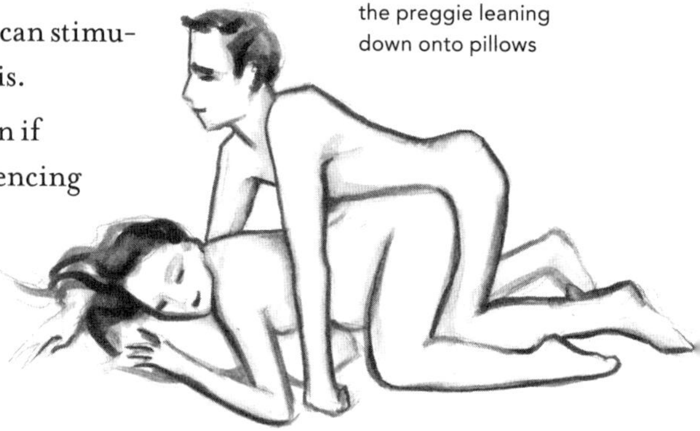

FIGURE 3.12
Rear-entry position with the preggie leaning down onto pillows

Variations include:

— Leaning forward onto pillows (see Figure 3.12).

— Bending over the bed, using pillows as support, with your lover standing and entering from behind (see Figure 3.13).

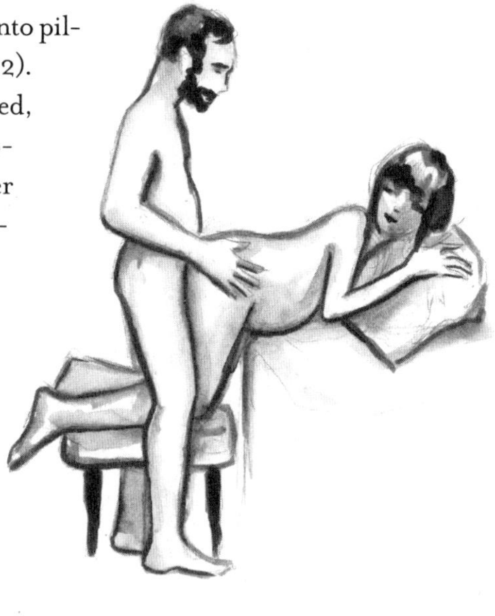

FIGURE 3.13
Rear-entry position with the preggie bending over the bed and her lover standing and entering from behind

Standing

Both of you stand upright, with your partner entering you either from the front or from behind (see Figure 3.14). You can lift one of your legs and turn it outward so your lover can enter you more easily.

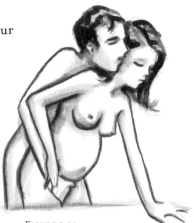

Benefit of Standing

~ Your lover can clasp and play with your breasts.

FIGURE 3.14
Intercourse while standing

Sitting

Have your partner sit in a chair or on the edge of a bed and straddle him or her (see Figure 3.15). Draw yourself up against your beloved's body and move up and down on his erection or her strap-on. Or lean your body backward, allowing your partner to take the lead in the thrusting motion.

FIGURE 3.15
Intercourse
while sitting

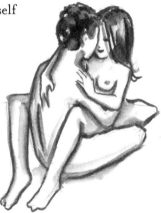

How You Can Help Her

To help prepare her body for delivery, practice massaging her perineum, the area of soft tissue located between her vaginal opening and anus. This will not only help to lessen the stinging sensation she'll experience during crowning, but will also make it less likely that she'll tear or need an episiotomy on D-day—two conditions than can really put a damper on postbirth sex. To begin your perennial massage, grab a nonirritating lubricant and spread her legs as wide as is comfortable. Slide your thumb into her vagina as deeply as you can. Now press down with your thumb, toward the rectum and sides. She may feel a slight burn or tingling from the stretch. Do not let up (unless she wants you to); rather, gently massage the lower part of her vaginal canal, pulling the tissue forward toward the opening, as the baby's head will do during delivery. Also, don't be afraid to orally stimulate her nipples, which can provide some relief and even turn her on.

{ **for partners** }

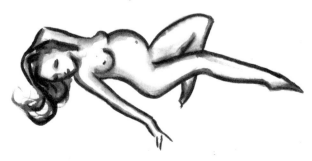

Benefits of Sitting

~ You can look into each other's eyes.

~ You can kiss more easily.

Variations include:

— Sitting on a chair with you facing your lover (see Figure 3.16).

— Sitting on top of your honey sideways (see Figure 3.17).

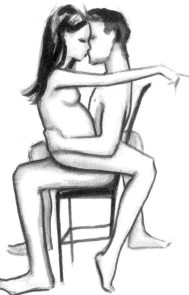

FIGURE 3.16
Intercourse while preggie is sitting and facing her lover

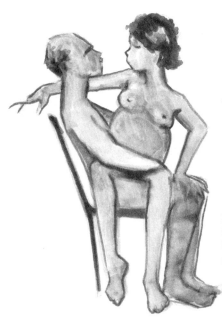

FIGURE 3.17
Intercourse while preggie is sitting on top of her partner sideways

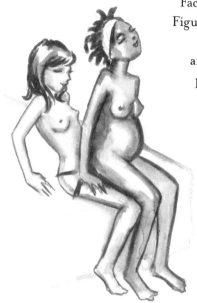

Facing away from your lover (see Figure 3.18).

You can also sit in an armchair and wrap your legs around your partner, who is kneeling in front of you (see Figure 3.19).

FIGURE 3.18
Intercourse while preggie is sitting and facing away from her lover

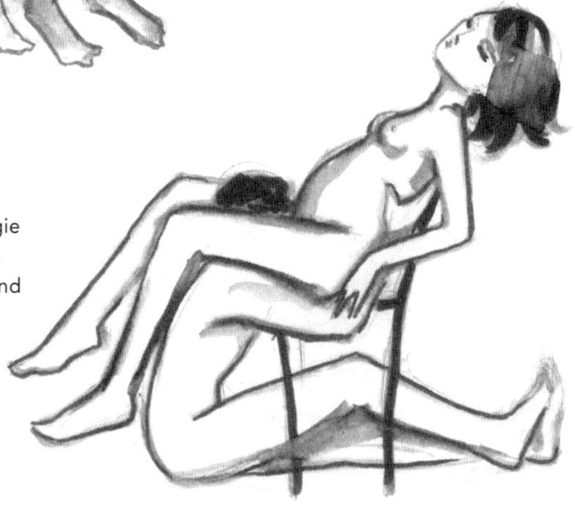

FIGURE 3.19
Intercourse while preggie is sitting in a chair and wrapping her legs around her sitting partner

You may want to sit on your lover's lap with the two of you facing a mirror for a full view of the hot action (see Figure 3.20). Or try situating your bum on the edge of the bed, then leaning back with your knees bent at the edge of the mattress. Depending on the height of your bed, your partner can penetrate you while kneeling or standing in front of your spread legs (see Figure 3.21).

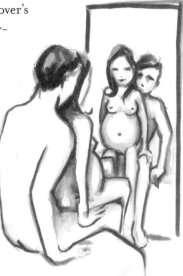

FIGURE 3.20
Intercourse while preggie is sitting in her lover's lap and both partners are facing a mirror

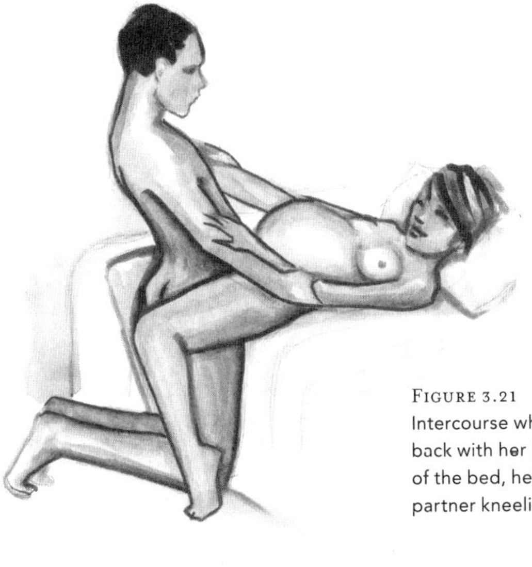

FIGURE 3.21
Intercourse while preggie is leaning back with her buttocks at the edge of the bed, her legs spread, and her partner kneeling or standing

☙ Hot Mama Kama Sutra

If you're experiencing more intense sexual desire, pregnancy may be the perfect time to explore ways to prolong and vary your love-making by practicing the teachings of the Kama Sutra. The Kama Sutra, an ancient Indian text dealing with love and sexuality, suggests activities like creating your own love chamber, focusing on kissing, and building sexual tension during hours of play. During pregnancy, the Kama Sutra advises lovers to concentrate on activities that stimulate a woman's vulva and perineum. It also encourages the woman's lover to regularly suck on her nipples, readying them for breastfeeding by "toughening" them up. Beyond the pregnancy precautions we have outlined, the Kama Sutra recommends avoiding positions that:

* ❖ are uncomfortable or painful

* ❖ affect a preggie's balance

When to Stop Having Sex

At any point in your pregnancy, Dr. Meulenberg advises that you should stop having sex if:

* ❖ it doesn't feel good

* ❖ you experience spotting/bleeding or unusual discharge

* ❖ you or your partner has an active genital infection

* ❖ you experience abdominal pain

* ❖ your health-care provider advises against it

———[**for hot mamas**]———

❖ require a woman to draw her legs across her abdomen or chest

We could devote an entire book to Kama Sutra pursuits during pregnancy. What we've included here is just a teaser to pique your curiosity. If you want to explore the Kama Sutra, we highly recommend the following two books: *The Complete Idiot's Guide to the Kama Sutra* and *The Supercharged Kama Sutra*.

𝔈 Epicurean Delights

Although pregnancy involves a number of restrictions against things that can go into your mouth (e.g., caffeine), fortunately a partner's genitals isn't on that list. This is great news, because intolerable vulval swelling may mean you're not always in the mood for sexual intercourse. When you or your partner longs to change things up a bit, or when you just want something to feast on, let your partner know that your latest oral fixation is on his or her body.

Interestingly, research shows benefits of fellatio during pregnancy. A 2002 study found that women who perform oral sex on their baby's father during pregnancy have safer, more successful pregnancies. This appears to confirm a 2000 study that indicated that swallowing semen during oral sex is correlated with a diminished occurrence of pre-eclampsia. (Pre-eclampsia, a condition that can occur in the final phase of pregnancy, involves an increase in blood pressure, possibly affecting kidney function. It can progress to eclampsia, which can involve convulsions, hypertension, and protein in the urine.) The Dutch researchers speculate that the reason for this effect is because the woman's immune system more readily accepts her partner's sperm with regular exposure to it. Because pregnancy disorders often stem from the mother's immune system rejecting the fetus as a "foreign body," her regular exposure to the father's "foreign proteins," which are also found in the baby's genes, will make her body likelier to accept them. Basically, the antigens found in his sperm can change her immune response toward the baby.

So, Hot Mama, if you can stomach it (and, of course, if his semen doesn't put you at risk for any sexually transmitted infections), it's high time to consider swallowing if you aren't in the habit already. It is believed that the protective effect of oral sex is strongest when a woman ingests her partner's seminal discharge. You see, aside from the fact that we're huge fans of head, we're really promoting it for the sake of a lower-risk pregnancy!

🐍 Worship Your Preggie, You "Cunning Linguist"

Tending to the luscious, throbbing, delectable lips between your thighs is a must. While there is, as yet, no scientific research promoting the benefits of a woman's vaginal juices on her lover's

WHAT'S GOING ON WITH YOUR PARTNER

According to research, a male partner can become closely attuned with a pregnancy, depending on whether he sees it as an opportunity for personal growth or a threat. Many men feel great during their partner's pregnancy. Filled with a sense of renewed potency, they enjoy the intensity and intimacy of pregnant sex. Some even feel that they are nourishing or "feeding" their partner and baby during intercourse, especially during ejaculation. Others experience heightened awareness before and after they've come, with increased physical and emotional sensitivity. Still others experience dreams and fantasies about intercourse, placing them in the role of giver to the woman's receiver. As previously mentioned, during a partner's pregnancy men may put on weight, feel gastric upset, experience toothaches and headaches, and even undergo phantom pregnancy. Pops-to-be can find themselves all over the map, just like the preggie herself!

{ for hot mamas }

health, ancient civilizations considered female emissions a sacred, health-inducing fluid. Witnessing a female ejaculation was actually a divine right of passage in many Near Eastern and South American cultures. Girls in some cultures weren't considered women until they could successfully "squirt the wall," thereby elevating their lovers to "official" manhood for having coaxed her to climax. (After centuries of being cloaked in misunderstanding and denial, a woman's ability to emit fluid during climax is once again being celebrated. Pregnancy can be the perfect opportunity to explore and realize one's ejaculatory potential, as pregnant women are known to ejaculate more readily. Check out Deborah Sundahl's *Female Ejaculation and the G-Spot* for more dish on getting wetter and better in the sack.)

Even if it doesn't lead to female ejaculation, cunnilingus affords a huge range of benefits for both partners. Whether it's the main event or foreplay, it can be just the sexual fix the two of you need without involving all-out intercourse. Oral sex can cause orgasm to occur more readily and intensely.

Pregnancy can alter some of the body's chemistry, which is good to be aware of if you're going to indulge in cunnilingus. Norton, a thirty-three-year-old papa of two, explains, "With our pregnancies, there has been no decrease in behaviors like oral or manual stimulation. There has been a difference, though, in secretions, like taste and smell. It's not bad necessarily. It's interesting, and I may have avoided oral sex at first because of it. But if I feel like it, I don't have a problem doing it."

We commend Norton for his willingness to oblige. Keeping your Hot Mama happy down below is an absolute must for reducing stress, staying connected, and taking advantage of the thrilling array of sensations this special time has to offer. No excuses, partners! Take after Norton, despite any change in taste. Have fun adding edibles, like flavored lube, if you must. The makeup of a pregnant woman's emissions may be altered dramatically in re-

---

WHAT'S GOING ON WITH YOUR PARTNER

Although thrilled with the pregnancy, your lover may also feel a bit jealous or displaced, especially if the two of you aren't doing enough bonding. Be sure to include your partner in your OB-GYN appointments. Give your lover copies of your ultrasound to carry around so that he or she feels more connected to both you and the baby.

─┤ **for hot mamas** ├─

---

sponse to dietary and hormonal changes, often resulting in a salty or metallic flavor. Still, the overall benefits of oral sex for Hot Mamas and their partners far outweigh any downsides involved in adjusting your palate.

In the latter portion of pregnancy, oral sex can offer a welcome change for any couple stressing about the constant focus on the enlarging belly. For partners having trouble overcoming the sight of the distended belly, Hot Mama's top half can be draped or covered. While your size still permits it, prop yourself up to get a full view of the action below, which will spike your thrill factor even more.

Warning! It is vital that partners of preggos *never* blow air into the vagina at any point during sex play. Blowing air into the vagina could result in an embolism (obstruction of a blood vessel), which can have harmful, even fatal, consequences for mother and baby. Embolisms can occur in nonpregnant women as well, so a "no-blow" policy must apply at all times during cunnilingus.

☙ Out-of-the-Ordinary Anal Pleasures

Oh, the pleasures of analingus! For those who indulge in the slightly naughty, oh-so-rewarding practice of oral-anal pleasuring, the unparalleled intensity of stimulation it provides often leads to ecstatic heights. Always practice care when you play in the highly delicate backdoor area, due to the risk of infection. Our recommendation: Use a latex dental dam or a barrier fashioned from nonmicrowaveable Saran Wrap. In addition, wash the area thoroughly with antibacterial soap prior to tonguing it down.

The anal sphincter and perineum are two of the body's most sensitive areas. If you've never engaged in any action involving these parts, now may be the time since it's one other way in which couples can be sexually intimate without necessarily "going all the way." You may get all the satisfaction you need from such delights, as the lovely Julienne, a twenty-nine-year-old mother of a toddler, discovered during her pregnancy. "The first time my husband put his mouth back there, I went wild," she says. "It was like a whole new bodily experience. My orgasm was so intense. I felt like a dirty girl doing something very taboo. Who knew that your rear was such a hot zone? It was thrilling and orgasmic. I cannot describe the difference in my orgasm, only that it was very intense and very delicious."

Research has found that most sexual experimentation takes place between the twelfth and thirty-second week of pregnancy, when more couples take advantage of the woman's heightened libido to expand their sexual repertoire. A 2000 study reported that many expectant couples change up sexual positions and try new caresses, fantasies, sexual games, and different forms of mutual pleasuring. We share this info because in spite of your growing belly it's important to stay open-minded and experimental during this precious time—especially as you head into T3.

🦢 Pregnancy Monsters, or Other Factors That Can Affect Your Game

It's important to know about other issues that can impact intimacy—things that aren't often mentioned in traditional pregnancy literature but that were brought up during our discussions with parents-to-be. Finding the time for sex, for example, was an issue highlighted by Chris, a thirty-something father who is launching his own company. "Sex is complicated because I'm doing a lot of traveling," he says. "So I just find that I've been taking care of my own pleasures. Sometimes it's easier to do that. If Pamela brings up sex, then I'll be totally into it. But timing has become more of an issue, especially since we're less likely to have a late night since she can be so tired. I feel like I'm in a holding pattern."

Chris's comments bring up the topic of pregnancy's love clock. A study of six hundred pregnant women revealed that most of them longed for their lovers between 10:00 and 11:00 A.M. and between 4:00 and 6:00 P.M. This contrasts with their nonpregnant counterparts, who typically preferred lovemaking in the evening and late-night hours. Ganem speculated that fluctuations in desire may correspond with a preggie's increased potential for hypoglycemia during certain times of day. Whatever the cause, meeting each other's needs can become more of a challenge with the change in a preggie's body clock.

Norton, whom we heard from earlier in the chapter, and his wife have had additional issues to deal with: "My wife is bipolar, so the only difference with our sex life during this pregnancy has been about medical changes with the prescriptions she's on, which can impact her mood. The hardest thing we've had to deal with has been safety for the developing child while she's pregnant and on medicine. We've been able to obtain absolutely no informational support on this issue, which is shocking. And that has had an effect on our relationship—the underlying level of fear and tension about the baby's health in general."

Lacking support during a pregnancy complicated by other medical conditions is a delicate and important issue, especially when there is no literature or media coverage available on the topic, and no support system in place. Couples may feel alone in their struggles, which can either bring them together or pull them apart. Many partners either turn to each other for support or withdraw from each other, with major consequences. If this is your story, make sure that you're not only leaning on each other, but also that you utilize your network, including any available support groups. If no support or advocacy group exists that deals with your issue, consider starting one yourself as a way to raise awareness, get and give information, and educate others about how to cope. Your little one isn't the only person growing leaps and bounds right now—you are, too! And you may be surprised at how much positive change you can bring about at this time in your life.

A preggie's bodily changes may leave some partners feeling less than enthusiastic. Allison says, "My breasts have made me feel strange and freakish. I don't think that my husband finds me sexier—he's more afraid. His view of me turns maternal, especially after our first baby was born, when being hooked up to a breast pump in front of the TV became my bosom's number-one purpose. The one thing that freaks him out during my pregnancies are my breasts—they're huge. My breasts are no longer a hot spot for him. He actually said to me the other day, 'They were perfect. What happened to them?' I was a D-cup before my first pregnancy, and funny enough, he prefers petite." Although some may question the sanity of Allison's husband for failing to love her luscious bosom, his feelings and opinions are totally valid and must be respected and dealt with. Discourse and disclosure can actually forge a stronger relationship if you're brave enough to go deep and deal.

Experimenting with new sex acts and new positions may make for some earth-shaking moments, but never discount the positive effect of small things, like changes in the frequency of your lovemaking and in how you define sexual intimacy. Many couples admit that they prefer abstaining from certain sexual activities while they're expecting. Every couple must find its own balance to meet each partner's emotional and physical needs. Simple acts of love, like cuddling and making eye contact, can keep you connected. So can communicating deeply, even when there are no major issues at hand.

Talk about your dreams, concerns, worries, and thoughts; share your joys, fears, sorrows, and excitement. And, Hot Mama, for heaven's sake—initiate! As Chris says, "It's important for everyone to be willing to put themselves out there, and it's more important for the woman to do so, especially if she's with a man who is considerate of his partner. Pamela has all of these changes going on and doesn't always put it out there that she wants to make love, and that makes me less likely to ask. Pushing sex is a double-edged sword. When we do it, it's great—it's very pleasurable and loving. If my partner is into it, then I am."

Here's a bit of advice that bears repeating: Don't forget to touch each other as often as you can throughout the day. Simple, affectionate, nonverbal gestures like kissing, caressing, and hugging can do much more to forge a tender, trusting intimacy than any romp session.

[4]

Third Trimester Sex: Improvisation Is Key

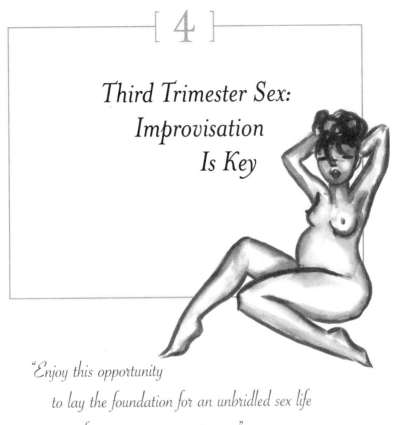

"Enjoy this opportunity to lay the foundation for an unbridled sex life after your pregnancy is over."

*Y*ou are likely to be a preggie-sex pro by the third trimester, particularly if you've been keeping things hot by following our recommendations. Still, looking down at a fetus in utero doing somersaults and making your belly dance can deter the staunchest Hot Mama from her sexy routine. Handling this third-party presence may define sex during your third trimester (T3). Fetal movements may diminish as the baby grows and takes up more room, but at the same time any movement is more noticeable from the outside. Activity cycles increase in length as D-day nears, but so do your babe's rest phases. Julienne, a film producer, says:

> I can recall that once, during a female-dominant sex session, the baby started doing what felt like flips. My belly was bouncing to and fro with increasing vigor as we tried to finish before our laughter took over. Thankfully, we were able to quell the giggles long enough to switch to a spoon rear-entry position, which allowed for climax. However, in later instances, we became too giggly and a bit unnerved by having the little one in such close proximity to our lovemaking. We resigned ourselves to spoon position only until the big day, when Papa happily hopped on top in an effort to induce labor. That time, however, it was Mama who couldn't perform.

The massaging action provided by sex-induced uterine contractions is actually good for the baby, as is the oxytocin dose you'll both receive during sex play, so cast all worries aside and get down to business.

✷ T3 and Your Sex Life

No matter what went on during the first six months of your pregnancy, the third trimester, defined as the period from the twenty-eighth week of gestation to delivery, may find your libido taking a serious nosedive. As your abdomen becomes increasingly crowded with baby and your organs scrunch closer and closer to your throat, feeling sexy can be a serious challenge. Along with tender, swollen (though magnificently plump!) breasts, the fatigue of toting extra weight can further reduce sexual interest and satisfaction. That's not to say that feeling in the mood is impossible. Many a Hot Mama is ripe and ready in T3, enjoying sex right up until she meets her child face-to-face. Making the most of whatever situation you find yourselves in comes down to your own and your partner's needs, desires, abilities, and preferences.

Don't for one minute think that you're anything less than a Hot Mama, regardless of what's going on. You are, quite literally, bursting with sexuality, from breasts to belly to booty. But if you find yourself getting lazy with the loving, consider that in 1988 researchers found that when both partners in a heterosexual relationship enjoyed sexual activity during pregnancy, compared to couples who didn't share mutual sexual joy, the relationship was evaluated more positively four months after delivery in the areas of tenderness and communication. Furthermore, three years later these relationships were evaluated as more stable and less affected by the pregnancy and delivery.

Not surprisingly, T3 keeps the woman's body extremely busy, especially when it comes to her sex organs. Strong vasocongestion in the genital area continues in months seven through nine, with or without the influence of sexual excitement. Vaginal orgasms, which may require an extra measure of forbearance and tenacity to achieve, can result in slow, thick waves of pleasure that surge through your weary body, restoring and rejuvenating it. Sure, difficulty finding and maneuvering into a comfortable position may make getting there a challenge, but the result is worth it. For those of you who find vaginal climax virtually impossible, clitoral orgasms tend to be a lot less challenging. It's a great time to bust out the vibrator or to employ finger tricks. If you feel grateful for anything at this point, it will be the speed with which you can reach clitoral climax, thanks to that occasionally bothersome engorgement!

If you cannot climax at all during T3, don't panic. The same is true for at least 20 percent of women. Bear in mind that the expansion of your abdominal muscles in every direction can render virtually unattainable the muscular spasms of orgasm, which can lead to the buildup of a frustrating amount of sexual tension that never ends in climactic release. For those of you stuck in plateau land, be assured that our Kegel routines will have you back in orgasmic action fairly soon postpartum.

Plenty of Hot Mamas in the middle of T3 report a continually expanding sex drive and thoroughly enjoyable sex life. They are determined to do whatever it takes to keep themselves feeling sexy and radiant. Harnessing your power, taking charge of your body and pregnancy, and choosing to enjoy the experience can help you keep your glow up. So can believing that you deserve and

WHAT'S GOING ON WITH YOUR PARTNER

Research from 1996 found that male sexual interest remains mostly unchanged until the end of the second trimester, when it decreases sharply. Most men show more sexual initiative than women before, during, and after pregnancy, which is particularly interesting when you consider that popular belief holds that men have more hang-ups with pregnant sex than women do.

—[**for hot mamas**]—

can have sensual happiness and satisfaction during and after your pregnancy. Learn to be intimate with yourself by touching your belly, admiring it appreciatively from all angles and marveling at the wonder of it all. When you are able to embrace the magic of the new life within you, you become empowered to experience the heights of pleasure and satisfaction. Radiating life, love, and fulfillment translates into more intimacy and closeness with your partner. Loving your pregnant body is the Hot Mama's secret of self-love.

We realize that the latter part of pregnancy can often be defined by weight gain and other inconveniences that conspire to test just how sexy you feel. In addition to a constant clitoral erection, many women experience occasional to frequent muscle spasms, which can be unnerving because they are difficult to differentiate from Braxton-Hicks contractions and early labor, especially for first-time mothers. Braxton-Hicks contractions before or after climax, sometimes lasting up to a half hour or more, are perfectly normal during T3. As mentioned in an earlier chapter, these muscle spasms can result from extra blood in the woman's genitals, emotional concerns, or prostaglandins in her partner's ejaculate. If uterine contractions are bothering you, one possible solution is to consider asking your partner to use a condom, or practice the withdrawal method. Either strategy will protect you from the prostaglandins contained in his semen.

Third-trimester sex can be pretty amazing if you know how to tap into its potential. Use some or all of the suggestions in this chapter to lift yourself up and over the T3 doldrums. More than anything, we encourage you to focus on comfort and connectedness right now.

Though we certainly don't want you to spend too much time comparing yourselves to the Joneses, know that about one-third of couples continue having intercourse into the ninth month of pregnancy. Many more would be medically safe doing so, but opt out for personal reasons. We hope you will be like Ananda, who was still getting busy by month nine:

> Semen is full of prostaglandins, which ripen the cervix and help labor come a bit faster. By the time you're forty-one weeks pregnant, it doesn't matter how many pillows it takes, you want those hormones and you want them now so you can have your damn body back. So we had been having sex every night for a week, cautiously, and with pillows, and as a compensation for the medically ordered fisting, a.k.a.

perineal stretching. One night, my partner commented that I was looking weirdly less pregnant. I thanked him, and we went to it with a will. He said, in the middle of things, "Wow. You're really hot and tight tonight." My reply was unprintable, but happy. Later, in the afterglow, he asked me why it had seemed so different. "The baby has engaged and dropped into my pelvis." "So it's sitting lower?" "Yeah, right against my cervix." "Your cervix?" "Yup. Probably you were having so much fun because your penis and the baby were occupying the same place." There was a full thirty seconds of stunned silence. "I. Just. Fucked. My. Baby's. *Head*!" "You could think of it like that." "Ijustfuckedmybaby'shead!" "Well, yeah." After that little incident, my prostaglandin supply dried up. With our second child, he swore off penetration as soon as the baby dropped. Wimp.

Regardless of your partner's response, sex after the baby has "dropped" into the birth canal in preparation for delivery may be quite different from a typical pregnancy romp. While the drop may help you breathe more easily, it also increases pressure on the pelvis, rectum, and bladder, resulting in tingly, pinching, or numbing sensations. The increase in size of vaginal muscle fibers also constricts the vaginal walls, resulting in a tighter fit for Hot Mama and partner. This can lead to pleasure or pain, depending upon the individual and whether there's more than one fetus.

Such changes to a Hot Mama's body inevitably make for fluctuations in sexual desire. A study of 600 pregnant women found that couples may alternate between intense, frenzied sex and

WHAT'S GOING ON WITH YOUR PARTNER

Don't be surprised or take it too personally if your partner experiences sexual problems, such as premature ejaculation or erectile dysfunction, while you're in the family way. Decreased sex drive, reduced desire, and/or issues related to seeing you as maternal or adjusting to the baby can all shake up the game. In many cases, such issues will correct themselves during postbirth intimacy, so don't make a big deal of it. Simply be supportive of whatever is bruising your lover's ego or troubling his or her mind at this time.

─┤ **for hot mamas** ├─

periods of great tranquility when the baby and the impending birth are the focus. These quiet moments are a wonderful time for the family to connect and prepare for the future. Lovers should never assume that a partner's decreased desire for or abstinence from sexual activity during T3 is an indication of a problem. On the contrary, it's to be expected.

Expectant women in a 2001 study reported a decline in sexual activity as pregnancy progressed. The main reasons cited were poor or decreased health, less interest in sex, medical reasons for reducing sexual activity, medical advice about sex during pregnancy, and the ever-present stigma against getting busy with a baby mere inches away. A 2000 study of 141 pregnant women found that 58 percent experienced a decrease in sexual desire, vaginal intercourse, and overall sexual activity as pregnancy wore on.

How You Can Help Her

Clean the house! Research has found that when a partner frequently pitches in by mopping, dusting, washing dishes, and doing other household chores, the couple enjoys a happier sex life and better marriage. What makes these gestures such an aphrodisiac for gals? They demonstrate that their lover cares for them and understands their responsibilities. Don't forget, too, that your pitching in leaves her a lot more energy for putting out!

[for partners]

Felicity says, "By the eighth or ninth month, things are getting squished and your bladder is getting leaned on and it's not as enjoyable. I had no real desire at that point and figured it was perhaps my body prepping itself by making sure that nothing's moved around too much." Generally speaking, the preferred erotic and sexual activities of couples and singles alike tend to remain unchanged during and after pregnancy, though vaginal stimulation almost always decreases markedly in importance during the second and third trimesters.

Sexual Positions Best Suited for T3

For couples that are still up for shagging during T3, the ultimate challenge is often striking the proper pose. Finding and getting into a position that allows easy access and is comfortable (without triggering too much laughter!) can be challenging as the belly grows. The same safety precautions from early pregnancy apply during the third trimester. In addition, Dr. Meulenberg issues the following warning: "Late-term women should not be on their backs for long periods of time. It will compromise the blood flow to the uterus and placenta."

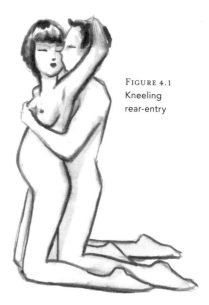

FIGURE 4.1
Kneeling
rear-entry

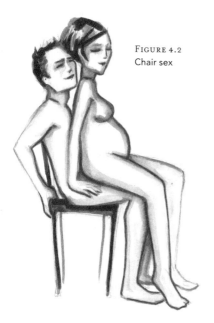

FIGURE 4.2
Chair sex

Bearing this in mind, we recommend the positions in Figures 4.1 through 4.6. The supported side-by-side position (see Figure 4.3) is a gentle option, and since you are on your side, a pillow can be used to support your belly. The woman-on-top position (see Figure 4.4) is recommended because it places no pressure on your abdomen, and you can use your lover's chest to stabilize yourself. Side-angle sex (see Figure 4.5 on page 110) is good if you are experiencing more sensitivity on one side of your vaginal vault. Supported by pillows, lie on your left side so as not to allow the inferior vena cava to compress under the fetus' weight). For more bodily contact, you can experiment with low-key loving (see Figure 4.6 on page 110). Since your legs are lifted there is less stress on your lower back, allowing you to relax more.

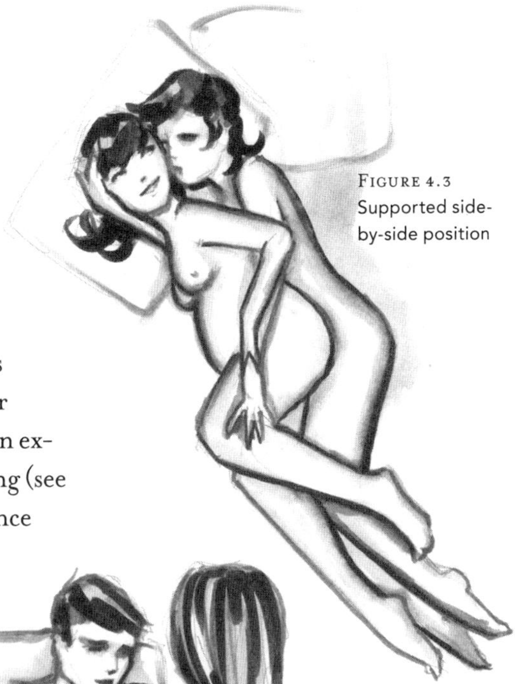

FIGURE 4.3
Supported side-by-side position

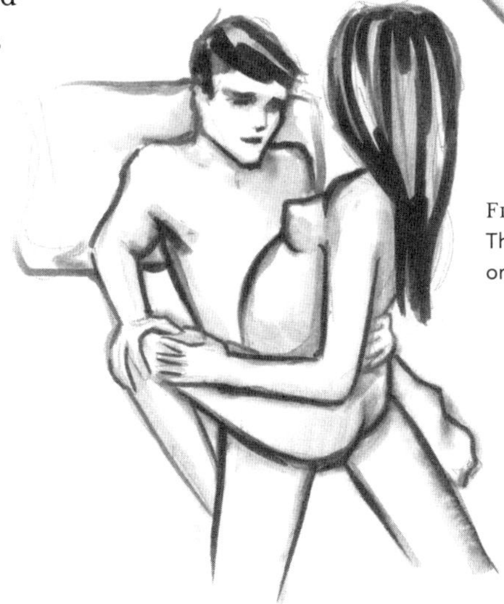

FIGURE 4.4
The classic woman-on-top position

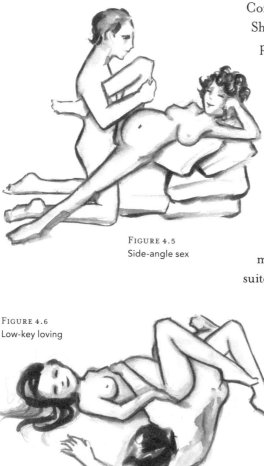

FIGURE 4.5
Side-angle sex

FIGURE 4.6
Low-key loving

Consider using Liberator Shapes to facilitate later-pregnancy sex. Liberator Shapes, found at www.liberator shapes.com, are billed as "bedroom adventure gear." They are padded supports that come in different shapes, and they help couples maintain positions well suited to lovemaking during pregnancy. Their contours provide additional support, reducing strain on hands and knees and making it easier for a pregnant woman's partner to maneuver around her belly.

How You Can Help Her

To orally pleasure her at any stage in late pregnancy, encourage her to sit on your face, or prop her pelvis up with pillows. These positions can help her relax, resulting in a much bigger payoff for your efforts.

┤ **for partners** ├

✿ Love That Lingerie!

Topping the list of popular positions during the third trimester, woman on top and doggie style tend to be the easiest for both partners. So saddle up or get down on all fours, but we want to see you flaunting your assets as you do so. Today's preggie lingerie styles offer more sexy options than ever. Sabine says, "The style today is really soft silk—not restricting, but flowy. When we got married, people gave me panties and open, flowy lingerie tops for sex during pregnancy. Yet they're comfortable to wear any time. Also, lots of the shirts that are now in style for going out can be worn whether you're pregnant or not."

An obvious and popular lingerie option for preggies is baby-doll style. Draping forgivingly over the belly bulge, these flirty and fun pieces highlight your breasts, buttocks, and legs, allowing both partners to (almost) forget about the baby for a while. Not all couples want to ignore the belly, though, as Raleigh attests: "I sometimes accentuate my belly in bed with some of the same lingerie as before, like a baby-doll cut. Pirro Cy thinks it's sexy. He's

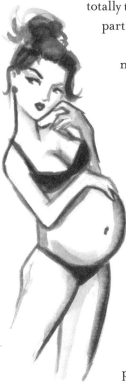

FIGURE 4.7
A preggie in
sexy lingerie

totally turned on. Me being the mother of his child is a part of that. We're more his now."

Riding high is the only way to go when donning your baby-doll fashions. Flaunting your voluptuous breasts above a flowing, sheer drape of fabric can help both you and your partner feel more comfortable and remain focused on the pleasure of sex play.

Variety is the spice of life, so be sure to spoil yourself with an assortment of belly-baring panties, hipsters, thongs, and bikinis (see Figure 4.7); check retailers like the Gap (www.gap.com), which has its own maternity line. Hot Mama bras come in silk, lace, minimizer, active, underwire, seamless, and double-strap versions, along with sultry garters and panties in bold leopard and other risqué prints, courtesy of our favorite teddy vendor Agent Provocateur (www.agent provocateur.com). Hanky Panky's fresh and fun preggie offerings, found at various outlets, include lace thongs, boy shorts, and bikinis.

Once you choose your look—or two or three—take your fun to the next level. Don lingerie that makes you feel like a diva, go heavy on the eyeliner, rouge, or lip color, lube yourself up with body oil, and throw on those f.m. heels that you never get to

How You Can Help Her

Your oh-so-pregnant partner may fear being incapable of satisfying you sexually. Know that both of you can achieve plenty of satisfaction during this awkward stage of pregnancy with a little patience and communication. Please, partners, if you are not already in the habit of doing so, let your preggie know how amazing it feels to be with her, to be pleasured by and to please her, and how much you love her. Terms of endearment and tender nothings murmured in vulnerable moments are wonderful lead-ins to all the pleasures we've been describing.

[**for partners**]

wear anymore, if only for five minutes and on your back, with the heels pointed upward! True, you may not be in the mood to impersonate the hottest porn stars or nude models, but take advantage of this unique time in your life to snap some erotic photos of yourself in all your pregnant sexy. Nude black-and-whites of you are classics you'll treasure forever. Hey, if they turn out awful or too racy for your tastes, you can always delete, burn, or let your snooping child destroy them later. Here's Allison: "I remember once, as a kid, I found this picture of my mother lounging back on a couch—naked and pregnant. I was horrified and ripped it up. I couldn't believe she did that. Now, as an adult and preggie, I wish I hadn't done that. She looked beautiful and it was such a wonderful image of a pregnant woman feeling good about herself. And based on other things she's shared with me about that time in her life, I think my parents really enjoyed the pregnancy phase, and that picture was a nice reminder of that."

🦚 Fantasy

One of the most tantalizing things about dressing up in lingerie and other sexy attire is that it can allow you to take on different identities and to play out fantasies. Fantasy and role-play work well, both in and out of pregnancy, to transport lovers out of their mundane reality and

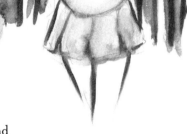

FIGURE 4.8
Dressing up can be a fun way to involve fantasy

into a lusty mindset. They can also serve as a powerful impetus to propel you out of a sexual rut.

If you think dress-up and role-play may be too extreme for you, know that there is a wide range of options to explore, from the tame to the hardcore (see Figure 4.8). We can pretty much guarantee that you'll find a comfort zone. If your fantasies seem too far "out there" or potentially offensive, use the trademark "I'm pregnant" excuse, and toss the blame on your hormones. Enjoy this opportunity to lay the foundation for an unbridled sex life after your pregnancy is over, especially if you've been apprehensive in the past about telling your partner your most unabashedly scandalous fantasies. Freed by the fact that you're "crazy" with child, any scenario goes. Let your lover see how "dirty," "freaky," or "kinky," you can be, then blame your hormones for your triple-X desires. Explore forbidden territory while you can get away with it!

Used properly, fantasy can arouse lovers to climax with surprising intensity and speed. It can help them to overcome anxieties and hesitations, explore new sexual outlets, and gain sexual confidence. Just think—no matter how you're feeling or what your pregnant body looks like, fantasy can make you utterly attractive, sexy, powerful, and maddeningly desirable. The element of imagination in fantasy can do wonders for boosting your self-image; the efficiency with which fantasy does the trick can spare your energy.

We came up with some fantasy scenarios to fire your and your lover's imaginations. Peruse the list by yourself or together. Expand on or alter our suggestions to suit your own tastes and proclivities. With the application of a little creative energy, we guarantee that you'll be dreaming up saucy scenes of your own before long!

1. Pretend that you're sexually inexperienced, and that you have no idea how you became pregnant. Tell your partner you know that you must've been a "bad girl," then ask your lover to show you how this might have happened to you. Let your partner act out the whole scenario, step-by-step and hands-on, to show you exactly how bad girls get knocked up. Play dumb the whole time, repeating that you just don't quite get it. Could your older, wiser teacher show you again? Play shocked and innocent, but moan in pleasure because it feels so good.

2. Pretend you're a pregnant prostitute with a ravenous sexual appetite. Demand that your partner satisfy your insatiable sexual desire, telling him or her how and where you like it, and what you'd like to do to them. Even though you're the one being paid, how can a client refuse the needs of a preggie? Care to shake things up a bit more? Pretend you're a knocked-up nun and your partner's paying you retribution for having broken your vows. Spankings, anyone?

3. Imagine that you're Mrs. Robinson and your partner is a hottie of barely legal age whom you can't resist. Show your lover the way a real sex pro does the deed. Give samples of your most advanced tricks, teasing and titillating until your partner begs for relief. Then, demand to be satisfied. Show your partner different techniques and positions as though they've never seen or heard anything of the sort before.

Flaunt the fact that you're already knocked up as evidence of your expertise.

4. Be the preggie porn star we mentioned earlier. Talk dirty the whole time. Say, "Mommy can't wait to have your dick," or "Mmmm, this preggie princess is craving your cream," or "Give my hot pussy your stiff cock," or "I'm totally strapped up and stuffed—can't wait to fill you," or "Now that you've knocked me up, you need to tie me down," or "Ooooh, this preggie plaything needs to be punished." As you can see, the possibilities are endless—*if* you surrender to your inner porn star. You may want to rouge your nipples and wear more makeup than usual. Paint your nails a racy shade of red or black and really vamp it up. Wear a garter belt (no panties) under a lacy baby-doll top, and don your slutty stilettos. Try taking your partner's penis between your feet or fingers with their dark, enameled nails, "threatening" his member (playfully, of course) with those painted talons. Your red, lipsticked mouth around his cock has the same effect. And don't forget to swallow! You are a porn star, after all.

Speaking of porn, even if it's typically not your thing, tons of print, online, and video pornography showcases the babe with baby. When *Hustler* magazine was in production, practically every second issue featured a pinup of a hot, ripe mama shaving her swollen vulva, tied up like a sex slave, practicing discipline dominatrix style, or getting down with a vibrator, daddy, or lesbian lover. Although the images of them are computer-enhanced (as is the case with any centerfold model), these playmates of pregnancy are great examples of positive portrayals of sexually attractive and active preggies—and inspiration for you to stay in full swing!

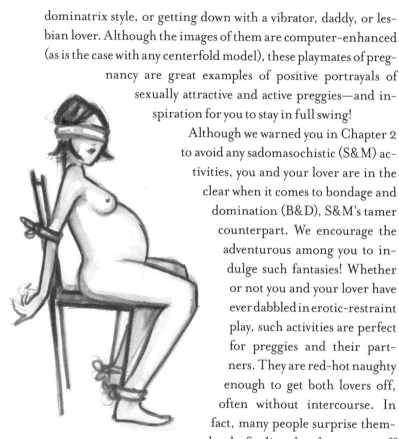

Although we warned you in Chapter 2 to avoid any sadomasochistic (S&M) activities, you and your lover are in the clear when it comes to bondage and domination (B&D), S&M's tamer counterpart. We encourage the adventurous among you to indulge such fantasies! Whether or not you and your lover have ever dabbled in erotic-restraint play, such activities are perfect for preggies and their partners. They are red-hot naughty enough to get both lovers off, often without intercourse. In fact, many people surprise themselves by finding that they can get off solely on naughty acts of playful aggression, including biting, being tied up (see Figure 4.9), or being "forced" to satisfy a dominant lover's sexual desires.

FIGURE 4.9
A preggie tied up
with bondage tape

WHAT'S GOING ON WITH YOUR PARTNER

Your honey is also experiencing libido changes. He or she may be more turned on or totally turned off by your pregnancy. In the case of the former, part of your partner's excitement has to do with the fact that he or she is having sex with a "different" woman. The newness of the experience, whether it's because of how you feel or how you look, can really get your partner off. Join in by playing up the mystery. Lose yourself in the fantasy of naughty seductress or dirty little housewife, and get free of the "But I'm a mama" mentality. Pretend your partner really is making love to another woman, one who's a bit Lolita "bad." Cut loose, have an out-of-body experience, and let your imagination run wild.

[**for hot mamas**]

🌿 Carpe Diem

Massages and cuddling can provide a heightened sense of intimacy during T3. Use touch techniques to stimulate your senses, keep you connected with your partner, and increase waning desire. Stoke the flames of passion with scented candles and other ambiance enhancers. Aromatherapy oils infused with rose, lavender, geranium, chamomile, or spicy scents are wonderful additions to late-pregnancy massages. A good massage not only relieves tension, stress, fatigue, and pain, but also can help the growing fetus by eliminating toxins from the mother's lymphatic system.

Regardless of how you choose to spend it, savor this precious last bit of time alone with your partner. It will be at least eighteen years until your full autonomy as a couple returns! Sabine says, "Throughout the rest of our life, finding time for lovemaking will be a challenge, so we need to cherish the time we have with no other things going on."

Obviously, you should never have sex if you really don't want to. Bow out with a polite "No thanks" or "Not this evening," without guilt. And know that your partner has as much right to refuse as you do. Raleigh handled her husband's opting-out gracefully. "Ever since the thirty-six-week mark, when the doc could feel the baby's head with his fingers, Pirro Cy said he wasn't coming near me. It's now a nonissue. Sex doesn't happen. Yet we're closer than we've ever been, intimate through touch, cuddling, petting, kissing. He'll sit there in my arms and I'll caress him or kiss him."

In your sex life, as in everything, honor your true self and your heart's desires. However, don't forget to entertain the possibility of using sex to expedite delivery. Research indicates that sex may actually make D-day happen much more quickly and smoothly. Read on.

❦ Sex Near the Time of Your Due Date May Help

With all the mixed information floating around concerning sex near your due date, we need to set the record straight. Prostaglandins, which are chemicals present in male semen, are widely believed to aid in the induction of labor. For years, midwives have suggested topical application of semen to soften the cervix and help it ripen. And as we discussed in the last chapter, some research indicates that swallowing her partner's ejaculate during fellatio can actually be good for a pregnant woman and her baby. "I encourage my patients to have lots of sex in the last month," says Dr. Meulenberg. "For some it works, for others not."

What about fears of triggering a premature birth? A 2001 study involving nearly six hundred women at three prenatal clinics found strong evidence *against* the popular notion that sexual activity correlated in any way with increased risk of preterm delivery. Continuing sexual activity into late pregnancy was actually a strong predictor of the pregnancy's going full term or beyond. While researchers could not identify the mechanisms at work, their findings turned up evidence that late-pregnancy orgasm, even in the absence of intercourse, reduced the risk of preterm birth. Other studies have confirmed similar findings.

A 2006 study involving two hundred healthy women with uncomplicated pregnancies found that among overdue births, the sex "home remedy" is safe and effective. Women who had intercourse late in their pregnancies (about four times a week from the thirty-sixth week on) were more likely to deliver between the thirty-ninth and forty-first week than those who abstained.

Sex appears to be a natural way to jump-start labor, though most of our physician friends remain unconvinced that the relationship is clear-cut. We are certain, however, that the prospect of late-term sex usually thrills couples, especially the woman. Most women, eager to reclaim their bodies, are totally up for evicting their little tenant by the end of T3.

Dealing with leaky boobies? Nearly every woman we interviewed noticed some breast leakage by pregnancy's end. Phasing into the third trimester, breasts tend to leak a little colostrum, a usually yellowish, although sometimes clear, fluid that is high in protein, carbohydrates, and antibodies. Colostrum is designed to nourish your infant during the first couple of days following birth. Nipple massage is especially beneficial during this time. It helps you prepare for nursing and also promotes the release of the mood-elevating neurotransmitter oxytocin, sometimes called the bonding hormone. Close to your big day, nipple massage can expedite labor and the oxytocin-exchange cycle. To induce labor, you and/or your partner should rub and massage each nipple and areola for fifteen minutes, three times a day. You'll feel your body relaxing more with each session.

☙ Not-Quite-Intercourse Options

Because many couples may not be up for sexual intercourse during T3, we want to be sure you have a number of alternative methods for staying connected during the last totally private moments you and your partner will have for a very long time. A wide array of options exists to keep your action hot and thrilling.

Interfemoral Sex

When your energy's tapped out, a good option is interfemoral (literally "between the thighs") sex. Your partner thrusts a dildo or penis back and forth between your lubed-up thighs while the two of you maintain full-body, skin-on-skin contact. This action can spell divine relief for a throbbing vulva, raging clit, and pulsating penis. For the highest degree of stimulation to both parties, squeeze your legs tightly around the phallus and vary the amount of pressure you apply.

Fleshlight Fun

When you're not in the mood for all-out intercourse, hand your lover a fleshlight. Hailed by countless men as the ultimate male masturbation toy, this soft, silky, penis sleeve replicates the feeling of a vagina. It resembles an oversized flashlight in transparent casing, but the lid at the end twists off to reveal a realistic-looking "vulva." It has a removable base for those who need greater length or who want to insert a vibrator. This toy, made of phthalate-free "reel-feel super skin," will keep him happy while you a get a break.

Bondage Tape

Kink it up a notch by mummifying each other with bondage tape. Made of thin, colorful, plastic material, this two- to three-inch-wide tape makes for a perfect blindfold, erotic gag, or bind. Create new looks by "dressing up" in the tape, use it to bind your love slave's ankles and wrists, or wrap a few key spots and snap some sexy photos.

Autoerotic Access

Don't let that belly get in the way of your self-loving. If your tummy is making it tough to reach your privates, try rubbing or squeezing your thighs together tightly. Reach down and around the belly for side-entry access, or boldly go around the backside. Stimulation from alternative angles can be challenging, but it's well worth it. If you have a sensitive anus, a round-the-back routine will stimulate additional nerve endings in your backdoor area, enhancing your pleasure. Better still, lengthen your reach with a vibrator. It's sure to get you off quickly and easily, saving you a lot of work. Some preggies experience their first "mechanical" orgasms during late pregnancy, with rave reviews (see below). As always, be sure to squeeze your PC muscles in tandem with your stroking, and get your workout as you work one out.

Sixty-Nine Me

Oral enthusiasts will particularly enjoy the benefits of the "69" position during T3. You will probably be most comfortable lying on your side. Using pillows, arrange yourselves into a position where both partners can simultaneously deliver hot tongue action, leisurely or frantically lapping, pressing, or massaging away.

😊 Your Battery-Powered Best Friend

That vibrating wand in the back of your panty drawer may become your best friend during pregnancy, even if you normally tend to shun manual or electronic masturbation. There's no better time than pregnancy to invest in a battery-operated sex prop. Your vulva, screaming for relief from the sexual tension caused by engorgement and the downward pressure in your abdomen, will thank you.

Favorite pleasure playthings of the pregnant set include:

✻ Waterproof Delight: a powerful multispeed vibrator that is perfect for private time in the bath or shower

✻ Mini or Pocket Rocket: fits into your purse or pocket for those on-the-go "emergency" situations

✻ Nubby G, Dolphin, UltraTech 3000, Rabbit: provide intense vaginal and G-spot stimulation via rotating shaft with the added bonus of clitoral massage from the base (girls, it doesn't get much wetter or better!)

✻ Venus Butterfly: can be worn like a G-string over your clitoris, providing you pleasure no matter where you are (as long as it's noisy) or what you're doing. The remote-control version allows you and your lover to trigger the toy from afar

✻ iBuzz: plugs into your iPod or MP3 player, allowing you to vibrate your way to a sexy fix anytime, anywhere, in rhythm to your favorite music

✻ Je Joue: moves to vibratory patterns from preprogrammed songs; the music causes the toy to twirl, swirl, quiver, and vibrate all over your body

✻ Clit Tickler: slides over his penis to rub its soft, knobby nodules against her clitoris during intercourse, providing both partners with great pleasure

✻ Erection Master: a flexible, vibrating silicone ring worn at the base of the penis to stimulate both partners' genitals

We have included the contact information for a number of reputable sex-toy retailers in the Resources section in the back of this book. Exploring the wonders of vibrator-induced euphoria can double the fun for couples, so choose one of the more advanced devices that titillate both partners simultaneously. Or take turns using a vibe on each other, hitting hot spots all over the body. These gadgets can stimulate much more than just the genitalia. If you use a toy for penetration in any orifice, be sure to apply plenty of lube.

Important: Never, ever swap sex toys with your lover until they have been properly cleaned. Cleanliness is an absolute must when using toys in the anal region. Pregnant or not, you don't want to contaminate your vagina with bacteria or viruses from the rectal region. If you must share, cover your toy with a disposable condom and change it with each use, or wash your toy with soap and warm water between uses. Even better: Spring for individual love machines.

🐛 Give That Preggie a Hand

Manual stimulation is a great way for your partner to pleasure you, no matter what trimester you're in or how big your belly is. A 1998 review of studies on sexuality during pregnancy found that 82 percent of pregnant women preferred mutual petting when intercourse had to be avoided for medical reasons.

Pregnancy can dramatically affect your tolerances and preferences, so be sure to communicate to your partner about how

---

HOW YOU CAN HELP HER

"Different strokes for different folks" is especially true during pregnancy. What felt good to your pre-preggie Hot Mama may now be too much or not enough. Flexibility, experimentation, and communication are key.

┤ **for partners** ├

---

much pressure you want and whether you want it applied directly or indirectly to clitoris, vaginal lips, and other sensitive hot spots (see the Appendix for illustrations of the female external and internal sexual anatomy). Using natural vaginal juices or your favorite lube, stroke her entire vulval area from anus to mons pubis. Zero in on the clitoris, lightly at first, then using firmer back-and-forth or circular finger motions, always checking in with her to make sure the pressure is just right. Once you've found the perfect touch, maintain a firm rhythm. Even if she started off wetter than ever, have some lube handy to keep things slick, smooth, and sensational for your sex goddess.

About two inches inside the vaginal opening on the front (stomach side) wall of the vagina lies the G-spot. This can be an incredibly arousing erogenous zone for women, especially during pregnancy—even if it wasn't previously. Venture just a little farther up, to the area between her G-spot and cervix, and you may be able to induce lots of natural lube by tapping her A-spot.

❧ The Keep-Him-Happy Hand Job

The simple deed of pleasuring him manually can be one of the best acts of love and generosity a tired preggie can bestow upon her partner.

Some happy variations to try:

❖ Slide the heel of your hand up and down the entire underside of his penis.

❖ Press your flattened hands against the sides of his penis and work your hands up and down his shaft.

❖ Alternating your hands, "milk" him with upward strokes from the base to the tip of his penis, or try the same in reverse.

Don't be afraid to use pressure; aside from getting kicked or punched in the groin, a man can actually handle a lot. And meanwhile, leave no hand idle and no other erogenous zone ignored. You can help him reach total-body orgasm by tending to other parts of his body while making his member the main attraction.

❧ Anal Play Without Going All the Way

Many couples enjoy anal pleasuring and make it a primary element in their sexual repertoire. One gynecologist reported in 1992 that 40 percent of preggies in his practice expressed a desire to engage in anal sex. If anal is a fave of yours but has become difficult during the third trimester, there are alternative ways to indulge. Gluteal sex and sex toys catering to the backdoor can offer an excellent way to pleasure your partner. See Resources for a listing of sex-toy retailers.

Important: When playing with any sex toy, but especially those designed for anal pleasuring, use a water-based lubricant that will not damage latex or invite infection.

Gluteal Sex

Some couples who find anal penetration too risqué take great pleasure in the almost-anal practice of gluteal sex. The thrusting partner uses the crease of the woman's buttocks (without ever penetrating the anus) as she contracts her gluteal muscles and rotates her pelvis to increase friction. Note: Lube is a must!

Anal Beads

Usually consisting of five or so plastic or latex beads that range in size from marbles to golf balls, strung together on a nylon or cotton cord, anal beads are ideal for easy stimulation of the nerve endings that line a lover's anus and rectum, or for giving your guy a delightful prostate massage (viva the male G-spot!). For those concerned with cleanliness, cover the beads with a condom knotted at the end. Using lots of lube—and we mean lots—insert the beads into your lover's rectum, one bead at a time, all the while teasing your partner's genitals to help him or her relax into pleasure and to intensify reactions.

Aneros

A secret weapon for advanced sexers, the Aneros is specifically designed to stimulate a man's prostate. Made of a nonporous material, it provides greater pressure than a dildo or vibrator can. Curled handles at the base press against the prostate both inside and outside of the body, adding even more sensation as he flexes his anal sphincter.

Butt Plugs

Whether rippled or smooth, large or small, butt plugs feel fabulous both on the way in and on the way out. Usually diamond shaped, with a narrow tip and flared base, butt plugs are usually offered in vinyl, silicone, or rubber. Silicone is our favorite, not only for its resiliency but also for its excellent ability to retain body heat—very important for user comfort. Furthermore, as the easiest of the three materials to clean, silicone can stand up to anal play's requirement for the highest standards of hygiene.

❖ ❖ ❖

Sex and intimacy during T3 will be what you make them. With the variety of options available to you, it's mostly a matter of choosing your preference. Be sure to maintain some sexual contact with your beloved, even if only by making suggestive comments during commercials while you watch TV. Even casually sexy interactions can keep your mindset primed for sensuality. Maintaining intimacy is paramount as you rewrite your sexual identities and repertoire during pregnancy to ensure that you and your partner will have an easier time adjusting to life with a new baby.

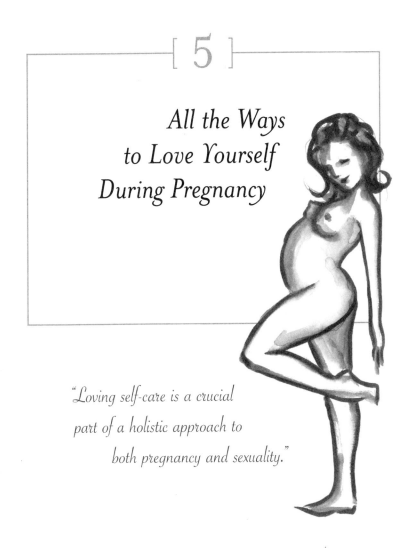

[5]

All the Ways to Love Yourself During Pregnancy

"Loving self-care is a crucial part of a holistic approach to both pregnancy and sexuality."

*R*egularly tending to your needs and inventing new ways to pamper yourself throughout pregnancy will increase bliss, reduce stress, and leave you feeling wonderfully sensual. Your sex life will benefit from a calm mind and a rested and healthy body—and so will your baby. Studies conducted in 2005 at Bristol University in England offered proof that controlling stress is vital for pregnant women. Cortisol, the primary stress hormone, crosses the placental barrier into the womb, immediately affecting your little boarder. Worse, late-pregnancy anxiety has been linked with elevated cortisol in ten-year-old children. Excess cortisol levels have been associated with immune suppression, weight gain, depression, elevated blood pressure, and a slew of other health problems.

Come with us, Hot Mama—we're about to show you how to kick the cortisol and kick into your sexiest self! The following suggestions are great for partnered bonding or solo time. We suggest you practice a blend of both, incorporating as many of these sensual secrets as possible into your routine.

For those who've never been much for self-indulgence, "stealing" some downtime may seem awkward at first. Sabine says, "I'm not big on pampering, but starting soon, I will go for massages. Somebody also suggested Reiki during pregnancy; they said it has a calming effect on the baby." She's absolutely right. Break out your schedule books and find some "you" time. Your overall wellbeing—and your sex life—depends on it.

How You Can Help Her

Ask her what you can do to make her life easier. Got kids? Offer to baby-sit. Run errands, do chores, fill her car with gas....

[*for partners*]

🐾 Walk This Way

For Danielle and a number of other preggies we interviewed, the simple act of wandering aimlessly around town, with no set destination or agenda, helped them tune into the body's subtle internal rhythms. Jill, Danielle's prenatal yoga instructor, used the following mantra: "You have nowhere to go and nothing to do." Embracing this mindset during a relaxing walk can help you release worry and stress. Spending quiet, sacred time with yourself in this way is a great balancer and soul tonic.

Are you at or past your due date? Walk your way into labor! Walking causes the baby to press down on the cervix, encouraging dilation.

🐾 Just Breathe

Do something most people take for granted—breathe! Relaxed deep breathing, known in yogic practice as *durga* breath, is an excellent tool for centering. Here are some guidelines from yoga instructor Paula D. Atkinson, who is based in Washington, D.C.: "Breathing in, first fill the belly, then the rib cage, then the throat. The breath should first be pulled down to the pelvic floor;

How You Can Help Her

Help your harried honey center herself by taking hold of her shoulders, looking into her eyes with a supportive smile, and asking her to breathe with you. Continue for a few minutes until she's calm. Finish with a long hug, and ask her what else you can do for her.

─────────────── [**for partners**] ───────────────

---

then it should fill the body from there, like you're filling a glass of milk. Next, empty the lungs slowly, from the top down. Release s-l-o-w-l-y. Making the exhalation twice as long as the inhalation can further relax you."

When you're looking for a quick pick-me-up, try the Breath of Fire, or Kabalabati. Atkinson explains, "These short breaths through the nose should start below the ribs. The short spurts of air shooting out through the nose occur from squeezing all sides of the waist in toward the middle." Kabalabati boosts your heart rate. It can also help mitigate the unleaded-coffee blues.

For either technique, do five to ten repetitions for optimal results.

❦ Know Your Acupressure Points

Tapping, rubbing, or pressing the acupressure points in and around your head, face, and neck is incredibly soothing (see Figure 5.1). It also enhances the flow of blood and energy that are fundamental to sexuality. Acupressure is an ancient Chinese healing art that encourages the body to rebalance its vital energy (its "chi" or "qi") by stimulating points along the energy channels, or meridians. Maintaining a smooth flow of chi can help keep your skin, muscles, organs, and emotions healthy, aiding in the prevention of disease and stress. For more information on helpful acupressure points I recommend Michael Reed Gach's book *Acupressure for Lovers*.

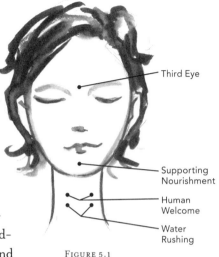

FIGURE 5.1
The acupressure points on the head, neck, and face

Third Eye

Supporting Nourishment

Human Welcome

Water Rushing

The stimulation of certain acupressure points should be avoided in pregnant women. John O'Connor, a massage therapist and owner of Rhythm Massage Studio in New York City (www .rhythmmassagenyc.com), explains, "Be sure to avoid the pressure point between the thumb and forefinger. Also, although you can rub your feet, take care to avoid pressing on the pressure points around the feet and ankles, as this can cause a downward rush of energy resulting in premature labor and other undesirable consequences."

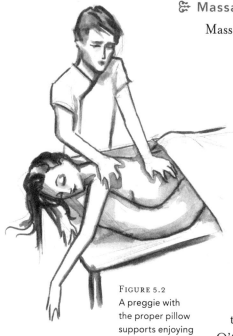

FIGURE 5.2
A preggie with
the proper pillow
supports enjoying
a massage

☙ Massage Is a Must

Massage makes you feel sexy! Prenatal massage loosens tight muscles, calms the nervous system, and increases circulation. Touch that is caring and sensually stimulating will coax you into a more positive, accepting mindset, enhancing bodily awareness and leaving you longing for love.

Aside from the obvious and commonly touted benefits of massage, it can also help deepen your connection with your baby. Here's John O'Connor again: "The baby is sensitive to the mother's emotional state. There's a lot of energy that comes into the baby. When a woman is constantly stressed out, the baby feels it. Massage releases endorphins and other good chemicals. When this happens, a person comes back into herself and heals. Things happen on an energetic level. A massage opens a gateway between mother and child. Instead of viewing the baby as an alien thing, she can connect with it. Massage puts people back into contact with their body and tunes

---

How You Can Help Her

Practice Hot Mama massage! A 2004 study exploring fetal-attachment behaviors, anxiety, and marital adjustment in American fathers found that those who learned to massage their pregnant wives improved anxiety levels and marital adjustment. This, in turn, affected paternal fetal attachment. Relaxation training was found to be even more effective than massage therapy.

Have her lie on her side, supported by pillows under her belly, and focus on kneading her shoulders, neck, thighs, hips, and buttocks. Work her scalp, hands, and feet, and alleviate muscle tension around her spine. For ideal support, try a prego pillow (www .pregopillow.com).

── **for partners** ──

---

them into what's going on inside instead of what's in their head. Massage is about coming back into your own presence."

Treat yourself to a good massage with an experienced prenatal massage therapist, preferably as often as your finances will allow (see Figure 5.2). Then coax your partner to imitate the techniques you've picked up from your professional masseuse.

During prenatal massage, unless you're physically and emotionally ready to initiate labor, beware of certain "hot" spots, specifically, those associated with bowel and intestinal release.

Massaging these areas can trigger downward momentum. Danielle recalls: "My water broke after an evening massage that followed a week of long walks, miserable prelabor symptoms, and utterly sleepless nights. My master massage therapist hit all of the "downward energy" spots with his magic hands, sending me into the most delicious dream state. When I awoke, my water broke and my baby boy was on his way. The benefits of massage are boundless and beautiful at any stage of pregnancy, provided you (and your massage therapist) know what you're doing."

Your massage therapist may integrate other bodywork or energy practices. Reiki, aromatherapy, the use of crystals and stones, chakra balancing, and other energy-stimulating techniques can enhance and deepen your experience, restoring balance to your chi and realigning your sexual energies to flow freely through your body. Hop your voluptuous self onto that massage table and see just how hot you can get!

Last but not least, reflexology, a specialized (and out-of-this-world) form of foot massage, is soothing to both you and baby. It can help with not-so-sexy pregnancy side effects like morning sickness, digestive distress, and lower-back pain.

🖋 Bath Time (Vibrating Rubber Ducky Optional)

Baths provide wonderful opportunities to relax, rejuvenate, and get into the mood. Accessorizing your bath time with candles or scented oils increases the sensual experience. Try eucalyptus, jasmine, chamomile, or lavender to promote relaxation; citrus or peppermint to invigorate your weary self when you're lacking pep; rose essence or rose petals to combat negative or distressing emotions.

🖇 Essential Oils Are Just That

Essential oils, indispensable for enhancing your bath or blending with an unscented massage oil, can alter your mood, appearance, and attitude. They can light your fire and soothe your soul. Lavender and myrrh are excellent for reducing stretch marks and improving skin elasticity. (Myrrh was a favorite of queens during pregnancy and birthing in Biblical times.) Avoid any essential oils designed to cleanse your intestines. They may cause diarrhea and can induce delivery. Oils to avoid are tarragon, rosemary, wintergreen, tansy (Idaho), sage, hyssop, calamus, and basil. Ones to use with caution include nutmeg, marjoram, eucalyptus, fennel, mugwort, celery seed, cinnamon bark, citronella, clary sage, and angelica.

🖇 Preggie Yoga

Prenatal yoga may be the single most beneficial practice you can add to your routine. It enhances your enjoyment of your body, boosts your spirits, and helps you reconnect with yourself—things that guarantee to enrich your sex life. Pregnant women must observe some precautions during yoga. Yoga instructor Paula D. Atkinson says, "Pregnant ladies should *never, ever* do twisting poses, and they should never lie down on the belly, even during early pregnancy. They should slow down their routine if they are used to doing a fast series of poses. I encourage them to pay close attention to the time of day the body craves movement. Finally, once a woman starts showing, she should always do Savasana (final relaxation pose) by lying on her side, in a fetal position."

Paula also cautions preggies to avoid any back-bending positions and inversions. Further, when doing poses like full lotus (see Figure 5.3), beware of the muscle-loosening effects of relaxin, a sex hormone that softens the pelvic girdle to allow for musculoskeletal expansion in preparation for labor and delivery. (It is the same hormone that makes some women physically more flexible during sex or during their period.) Elevated levels of relaxin increase the possibility of hyperextending the hip joints when performing certain yoga poses. Other joints (e.g., ankles and knees) may be a bit less stable, too, increasing your risk for twists and sprains, so be careful, Hot Mama. It's tough to feel sexy on crutches! Developing a strong abdominal core via yogic practice will alleviate some of relaxin's potentially problematic effects. A program for core strength that builds gradually will decrease the risk of injury while increasing overall bodily well-being. As a sexy bonus, tuning into energetic subtleties, exploring your musculature, and raising bodily awareness all deepen sensual pleasure and sensitivity.

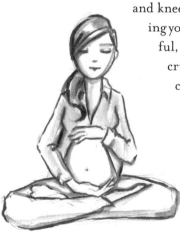

FIGURE 5.3
A preggie in full lotus position

🐾 Easy Exercise

Keep up your exercise routine during pregnancy to ensure that your energy level remains stable. Activities such as stationary cycling, hiking, low-impact aerobics, and swimming are fantastic choices for preggies. Invest in a good support bra and athletic shoes. Be sure to warm up before every workout, and keep your pulse below 140 beats and your body temperature below 100 degrees Fahrenheit. At the end of your session, take time to cool down and rehydrate.

Important: If you're pregnant, be sure to consult your healthcare practitioner before taking on any exercise routine, even if you're a veteran at working out. Be sure to stop exercising immediately if you experience dizziness, bleeding, trouble breathing or walking, irregular heartbeat, or pain in your back or womb while working out—and arrange to see a physician right away. Avoid exercises that involve contact sports or rough play (e.g., basketball, skiing, or waterslides), jerky movements (including some types of dancing), and being flat on your back.

🐾 Sleep Well

As your belly gets bigger, sleeping may become more difficult.

Rest is vital for overall well-being, sexual and otherwise. Try the following sleep-well techniques:

- ❖ Sleep on your side to allow more blood flow to the placenta.

- ❖ Cross your top leg over your body, placing a pillow underneath it.

HOW YOU CAN HELP HER

Get things done before she has to ask you to do them. This will help her feel supported and loved, which in turn will help her relax and be more sensual with you. Simple gestures go a long way, as Raleigh knows. "Pirro Cy would do things to prep for the baby, like installing the car seat," she says. "His taking the initiative to cross things off the to-do list has been so wonderful and has made things easier on me."

— [**for partners**] —

❖ To breathe easier, raise the head of your bed four to six inches.

ᕅ Music's Magical Effects

Musical vibrations directly affect your psyche, giving music powerful curative properties. Soothing tunes that have no lyrics are often best for mitigating stress and can be a great accompaniment to relaxing or doing yoga. Nostalgic, upbeat, and fun songs tend to elevate your energy levels. Pay attention to which tunes rev your engine and which knock you out. Play accordingly!

ᕅ Calming Colors

Pregnancy is a wonderful time to explore the effects of color. Experiment with different colors and textures in your clothing and linens to effect a calming response in your body's largest organ—the skin. For Danielle, luxuriating in new sheets with a higher thread count and a rich, sensual hue provided a major mood boost during the dark winter days of her pregnancy. Many preggies love crisp, cool, white sheets; others prefer a deep, passionate red. Whatever your preference, premium bed linens are an excellent way to splurge on your pregnant self.

🦋 Healthy Eating

Chances are good that you will wrestle with the weight-gain monster at some point during your pregnancy. Here are some effective techniques for warding off cravings when hormonal fluctuations and a rapidly growing fetus mess with your hunger cues:

- ✤ Eat your veggies and your protein.

- ✤ Keep a stock of healthy, well-balanced snacks on hand at all times. Good options include hummus or peanut butter spread on soy crisps, baked tortilla chips, or whole-wheat pretzels. Also try dry-roasted nuts, yogurt, chicken, fresh fruit, or energy bars.

- ✤ Eat whole, organic foods whenever possible, especially ones that come from the four basic food groups: protein, fruits and veggies, carbohydrates, and dairy products. Be sure to stay away from undercooked meats, unpasteurized cheeses, and deep-sea fish that may contain high mercury levels.

- ✤ Drink lots of water—at least two liters daily. Ironically, staying well hydrated helps prevent bloating.

❧ Take your vitamins. Pay special attention to your intake of folic acid and calcium.

❧ Stock up on quick-to-make meals to help ward off the temptations of fast food.

❧ Stay away from fruit juice and candy. Opt for real fruit instead.

❧ Eat small, frequent meals throughout the day, instead of three large meals, to ward off heartburn, indigestion, nausea, and "the bloats." Also avoid foods that are acidic, salty, sodium-filled, deep fried, or spicy.

❧ To promote good sleep, avoid chowing down just before bedtime.

❧ Pay attention to your body. Eat when you're hungry (not starving), and stop eating when you feel satisfied (not stuffed).

Remember, pregnancy is not an excuse to gorge yourself. A study from 2007 found that pregnant women who gained even the recommended amount of weight ran four times the risk of having an overweight three-year-old than the preggies who gained less. Your habits always come back to your babe!

Just as important, food choices impact how you feel, physically and emotionally. Regard this as a time to listen to your body and to eat intuitively; often your pregnant body wants the nutrients contained in certain foods, like bananas or spinach. When you feel a craving coming on, practice using the *durga* breath or distract yourself with some yoga poses. Here's Danielle: "My craving monsters were kept at bay only through preparation and forethought. Staring at the Taco Bell website, drooling to the point of tears, and telling my friends via e-mail and text message how *delicious* those pintos-n-cheese looked was not one of my prouder moments. Still, with all of my cravings for starchy foods, my weight gain stayed within the 'healthy' range of twenty-five to thirty pounds."

🦢 Sexy Preggie Style

Many preggies refuse to splurge on pregnancy attire that will be worn for only a few months. Instead, they opt for oversized, frumpy clothing that's anything but sexy. Don't do this to yourself, Hot Mama! Do right by your bodacious body (and your psyche) and walk into any maternity store, where positive attention and compliments will surely be showered on you, and where staff will help you select chic and stylish fashions that are perfect for your form.

Prefer to shop from home? Plenty of online boutiques offer form-fitting, sexy preggie and postbirth styles, including dresses, suits, and jackets; fitness/workout wear; swimsuits; camisoles and lingerie; nursing bras; and rock-n-roll T-shirts and tanks. Here are a few of the website that are worth taking a look at:

www.glamourmom.com
www.lizlange.com (also at Target)
www.apeainapod.com

www.bellybasics.com
www.japaneseweekend.com
www.unbuttonedmaternity.com
www.noppies.com
www.babiesnbellies.com
www.figure8maternity.com
www.topshop.com

❧ Invest in a Good Pair of Shoes

Since we're talking about basics, let's cover your feet. Pregnant feet may swell one or two sizes, especially during winter, so having at least one good pair of roomy shoes is a must. Select flat or low-heeled shoes (two inches max), with good traction and adequate arch support and made of breathable material that won't trap moisture. Sore feet are incompatible with feeling sexy, so keep your tootsies happy!

❧ Love the Ever-Growing Skin You're In

Even if you're a self-loving neophyte, take advantage of the novel experiences and sensations afforded by spending nine months in a new, transformed body to become a master masturbator. Masturbation is a smile-inducing, pulse-increasing, endorphin-releasing, stress-relieving joyride *every* Hot Mama should take advantage of (see Figure 5.4). Self-pleasuring gives you a chance to get to know yourself all over again from head to toe. It also acquaints you with the best touch-me-there techniques for when you're with your partner. If you find yourself needing a boost in bed, know that masturbation can turn people into better, more confident lovers. Plus, loving yourself and your body helps you to become comfortable with your pregnant figure and sexuality. Finally, vaginal lubrication produced during masturbation normalizes your bacteria count, warding off yeast infections and other such conditions that can arise during pregnancy.

Preggies who find that their orgasmic potential has drastically increased enjoy masturbation as an alternative method of releasing sexual tension, affording their lovers time to recharge. Hot Mama Raleigh says, "I have had days where I could spend whole mornings and afternoons getting off."

Encourage your partner to indulge in some self-lovin', too. Ignore any fear that self-pleasuring can indicate waning regard for your partner. On the contrary, masturbation keeps your fires stoked, even as it alleviates stress arising from mismatched sex drives and hectic schedules. The Hot Mama masturbation mantra is: Take no

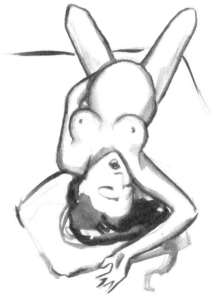

FIGURE 5.4
A preggie masturbating

What's Going on with Your Partner

Communicate about your masturbatory practices to prevent mis-understandings. Says Allison, "He's having trouble letting his needs be known. He's afraid to ask. And then our biggest challenge is finding the time. Going out on dates. There's too much other crap to deal with. We just have different perspectives on how to deal with his sexual needs. He's Catholic and I think that's impacting the way he sees me right now. But it hurts that he'd masturbate instead of trying to be with me."

Try not to be overly sensitive to the reasons your partner may have for going solo, for example, trouble making love to a pregnant woman because of negative religious messaging. Keep the door open for intimacy, but avoid forcing it open.

{ **for hot mamas** }

offense and accept none. Consult with your honey, like Sabine did. "If we have to wait for sex," she says, "then I'll be more than happy to masturbate or to let my partner watch porn while getting off. If it comes to that, it will be tough, because I'd rather be with my partner."

Eight to 31 percent of women admit to masturbating during pregnancy. Julienne says, "My favorite pastime around the fifth and sixth months became pleasuring myself. I must bashfully admit that the frequency of my masturbation sessions often exceeded

HOW YOU CAN HELP HER

Take your Hot Mama to the movies or out to dinner. Savor the time alone together while it lasts!

┤ **for partners** ├

two to three times per day. Between the weight of the fetus putting pressure on the nether region, increased blood flow, and raging hormones, I could hardly keep my hands off myself! The endorphin rush from masturbating helped me maintain self-confidence when my increasing girth made me feel like a whale."

Linger over the feel of your growing belly. Feel your body coming to life in so many extraordinary ways. Don't stop at one, Hot Mama—dare to become multiply orgasmic! Many preggies report breast-only orgasm for the first time during pregnancy. Don't miss your chance to join that club. Honor your goddess body. Get in touch with your genitalia.

🦋 Couple Time

Sweet, nonsexual delights shared with your partner can build tenderness, trust, and connection during pregnancy. One favorite activity is enlisting your partner in your personal-grooming regime. "I've tried to maintain my normal beauty routine," says Raleigh, "but the one thing that's gone by the wayside is the undergrowth, because you just can't see it. So Pirro Cy has tried to help me out with it."

Perhaps ironically, pregnancy can be a very lonely and frustrating experience, making a partner's support all the more important. Raleigh explains, "Pirro Cy has been so supportive by being involved in prenatal visits, reading with me, talking to friends about their experiences and then sharing them with me. We talk about the future and about parenting styles. He's showing how he'll be a good father, and it has increased my attraction to him."

Caring behaviors—whether bestowed on yourself or shared with your partner—tend to have that effect. Keep this chapter handy as a reminder of the many ways to pamper yourself during pregnancy. Hot Mamas know that loving self-care is a crucial part of a holistic approach to both pregnancy and sexuality.

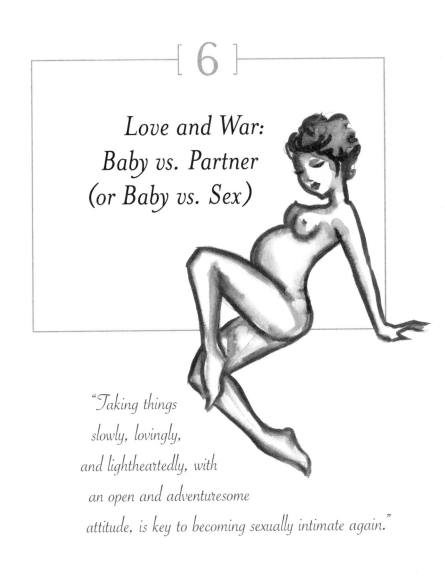

[6]

Love and War:
Baby vs. Partner
(or Baby vs. Sex)

*"Taking things
slowly, lovingly,
and lightheartedly, with
an open and adventuresome
attitude, is key to becoming sexually intimate again."*

*U*nderstandably, you're probably a wee bit immersed in your little one right now—and will be for quite a while. Eventually, though, you'll resurface from the joys of having a newborn, look at the other, much taller love of your life, and find yourself asking: Will we ever have sex again? This question haunts the hearts and minds of many new parents, especially during the physician-imposed "refractory" phase just after the birth, which can run from weeks to months depending on your delivery. If you're not careful, the time period following the Big Day can quickly turn into a subconscious war for your attention.

Many in our society know surprisingly little about childbirth and sex, even if they've participated in them. Add to this the fact that most of the literature on the subject of sex and pregnancy is sadly limited and far less frank than necessary for the establishment of healthy, comfortable discourse. Most couples lack the information that would help them rediscover and sustain a healthy sex life postbirth. Your Hot Mama mentor team wants to change that!

☙ Show Yourselves Some Compassion

When it comes to postpregnancy sex, the new mother's partner inevitably feels neglected by her, no matter how hard she has worked to prevent this from happening. Felicity says, "Sex postpregnancy is a very different situation. For about two months after giving birth, there was no way I was going to have sex since I was dealing with issues like exhaustion, hormones, and slight bleeding. The relationship became charged with a different intensity since I was now a mother focusing on her child. There was this shift in us because we now had another person, a helpless child, in the family."

The battle between baby and partner begins long before the little one's introduction into your life. The uncertainty that comes with knowing someone else is joining the mix can leave some partners, including the Hot Mama herself, insecure about the amount of attention and energy that will be left over for them. Unfortunately, regardless of good intentions on the part of either partner, both of you will be spread much thinner after your new arrival. Babies take a lot of time and energy, and there's no way around the fact that you will simply have less private time together. For this reason, it's very important to quell the trouble before it begins.

Probably the best advice we can give you about reclaiming everything in your life, including hot sex, is this: Don't push yourself too soon. It's unfair for anybody, including yourself, to expect too much of you right away. You have been through a lot physiologically, psychologically, and emotionally, so it is important not to overload yourself with too many activities, especially when it comes to pleasing anybody in your life who isn't "the baby." Draw your boundaries early to reserve your chi so you can expend it on the most important people in your life: your baby and your lover. Here's Felicity again: "It was such an exciting time, but at the beginning you cannot expect everything to always be 'tiptoeing through tulips.' It can be hard and isolating. Even though you have a newborn, you still need to do things with your partner alone, whether it's going out for dinner or out with friends. You need to maintain couplehood and not neglect each other. You need to stay connected because it's been such an awe-inspiring event and it can be easy to stay in on a Saturday night with your baby. It's okay to be away from your child and be with your spouse. It's key to do things together as a couple and maintain that bond so you don't lose sight of it."

❧ The Importance of Getting Laid

First, why do you need to have sex? To that we ask: Why not?

While you shouldn't need an excuse to make love, remember that sex is the foundation of your connection with your partner. Without it, you run the risk of becoming so detached as to barely recognize each other. Sex reduces stress and boosts your energy, and as any new parent will tell you, that's a good thing! The endorphins released during sex help you to feel more at ease and centered. This is something your baby picks up on. Your relaxed state ultimately helps your angel to sleep better and to be less agitated during waking hours. So give yourself permission to get intimate again. Have sex on a regular basis. After all, it's for the greater good of everyone involved. It's good for your physical, mental, and emotional health and well-being—all of which help to maintain a great family life.

Unfortunately, as mentioned, the lack of information and discourse on the subjects of postbirth vaginal healing in the new mom and libido recovery in both partners may drive a wedge between lovers, compounding issues. Most of the individuals we

WHAT'S GOING ON WITH YOUR PARTNER

A common complaint of new mothers is that their male partner doesn't seem to desire them anymore. A man may comment to his partner that he finds it hard to see her as a sex object now that she's the mother of his child(ren). Ask your partner if this has become an issue and how you can make sure that it isn't one. Then be sure to suggest ways your lover can support you in your efforts to step up. Furthermore, be aware that new fathers want their lovers to be sensitive to the additional stress they're experiencing. It can be difficult to feel excluded from things like breastfeeding. New dads, too, need to feel desired by the mother of their child, yet they are often hesitant to communicate their needs and are afraid of harming her during penetrative sex.

—[**for hot mamas**]—

spoke with said that they had not discussed postpartum sex plans with their partners, for reasons ranging from a fear of jinxing the pregnancy by thinking too far ahead, to an understanding that the birthing process itself can affect how soon couples get back into the saddle. Know that it is important for couples to touch base on the postpartum sex issue—and the sooner the better. With your partner, address your expectations, wants, fears, desires. Couples who don't have a heart-to-heart about such matters risk a breakdown in communication, resulting in an even greater fear of talking about these difficult topics and, ultimately, in a sense of isolation. You've already got enough on your plate; don't add a failure to communicate with your lover about postpartum sex to the list.

A study involving sixty first-time parents, all heterosexual, found that while these couples rated their relationship as highly harmonious during sex, there was a significant decline in marital satisfaction by the time the child turned one. Men were concerned about issues surrounding finances, leisure activities, and relations with family and friends, all of which became stressors in the love relationship. Wives wanted a lot more attention from their husbands than the guys were giving. The family climate had changed in the last year for both moms and dads, with increased distance between mates and a decreased experience of closeness for husbands. If the decision to have a baby had not been mutually agreed upon, or if one spouse had considered separation earlier, an even lower level of marital satisfaction was reported.

These sorts of statistics are fairly common (see the last section of the chapter). It's good for couples to be aware of them so that they can see how some conscious attention to their relationship can help prevent the gradual drifting apart. At the same time, don't let worry over your partnership infect your home life. Have compassion for yourselves as partners and as new parents.

🐚 I Want My Vagina Back!

The mere thought of getting back into the saddle after childbirth can provoke terror in the heart of a woman. *You wanna put that thing*

where? Depending on your birth experience, your vaginal opening may be too tender to even think about touching it for several
days or weeks afterward. Sex may be the farthest thing from your
mind. Or, worse still, the thought of being a kinky Hot Mama in
the sack may haunt your every waking moment.

The postbirth vagina is a great mystery to most men and
women. *Will it go back to normal? Will I ever feel anything there again?
Will it hurt? Is it stretched out forever? What can I do to get it back into
shape?* Your partner may also be very concerned about the condition of your vagina and about not wanting to hurt you. Frequently,
the partners of new mothers are scared to even broach the subject
for fear of seeming critical, or of causing unnecessary self-consciousness. They may secretly be unable to get the subject out of
their mind and may bring it into your sex life if you do not touch
on it first. So let's talk about that postbirth vagina.

As we've repeatedly stated, PC exercises are vital to the tone
and recovery of your vagina after childbirth. (Women who've undergone cesarean sections will also benefit during recovery from
the extra muscle tone provided by PC exercises.) If you have faith-
fully executed your exercises throughout your pregnancy, you really have little to worry about. Even small women with large babies
recover brilliantly with a little extra care. Your vagina may actually be tighter than it was before the baby arrived, given that increased muscle tone and time off from sex contribute to a tighter
fit. (This was the case for Danielle. See her story later in the chapter.) Continuing your Kegel routine and strengthening your

lower abdomen are keys to restoring your sex life to prebaby quality, even if the quantity has fallen off a little.

Vaginal strength aside, you may fear that having had an episiotomy incision or tearing will forever alter your nerve endings and pleasure zone. You may feel self-conscious about the appearance of your torn vagina and may actually grieve the loss of your "untainted" flower. On an emotional level, for many women, the first time they have sex after giving birth can be similar to losing their virginity. Your body is not the same as it was before you gave birth. You experience sex physically and emotionally as a different person, which can be exciting or scary, depending on any number of factors unique to every individual.

🦢 What Happened to My Body?

Your body is obviously very different from what it was before you became pregnant, so a fair amount of rediscovery is in order, for both you and your partner. You will want to explore yourself in private, especially as your belly slowly deflates like bread dough in the days following delivery. The strangest feeling is likely to be the initial shock of standing up for the first time sans baby as your organs do a dip. You will feel all sorts of movement in the intestinal region as things begin to drop back into place, most markedly on your first encounter with gravity. You mustn't allow the dough belly to make you feel less than sexy. Your tummy will be taut again in a few days. Think about the nine months it took to stretch your belly to that size in the first place, and allow yourself a couple days before worrying about flatter abs.

Understanding and accepting what is going on with your body without desexualizing yourself is very important to reestablishing a physical relationship with yourself and your partner. It is the rare couple who reports having no sexual problems after childbirth.

🦋 The Hot Mama Hiatus

Many women find themselves longing for affection from their lover within the first few weeks after giving birth. Others take more time. This is often directly related to the trauma or ease of the birth experience. "If you had an episiotomy, cesarean section, or other surgical procedure," says Dr. Meulenberg, "you may be on 'no sex' doctor's orders for longer than the six weeks recommended by most OB-GYNs and midwives." The bottom line is to do it when you're comfortable. There's no one right answer. If you're not ready, you're not ready, and that's okay.

Many people experience a mini identity crisis after the birth of a child, based on the concept of being a mommy or a daddy. Joining a new social rank is strange, wonderful, and frightening. You will never again be single and unattached! Your life of being responsible for only you is over. This can have sexual repercussions if you're not ready for it. In the meantime, make sure you and your partner plan for some serious cuddle time, with lots of hugging, kissing, and massaging. The same endorphins released during orgasm can be released in smaller doses by simple acts of affectionate touch. Don't deny yourselves any of nature's finest mood elevators. It's free and fun, so what have you got to lose?

Don't despair if after you've given birth your sex life isn't what it once was. Many postpartum women report a decline in sexual interest, libido, or desire. Universally, they will tell you that at one time or another they were too exhausted or weak to even think about getting turned on. "I wasn't even remotely interested in genital touch until about the fourth week," says thirty-eight-year-old Hot Mama Tammie, from California. "All of my energy went into the baby, no apologies."

Literature on the subject suggests that there are seven key factors involved in decreased frequency of sexual intercourse and reduced levels of desire and sexual satisfaction after childbirth:

1. adjustment to changes in the mother's social role

2. mood

3. fatigue

4. marital/relationship satisfaction

5. breastfeeding

6. physical changes associated with the birth of the child

7. hormonal fluctuation

Let's take a closer look at a few of these, and also at some other issues that may contribute to the situation:

❖ Vaginal soreness may last for several months, especially if you experienced tearing or underwent an episiotomy.

✤ Levels of the milk-production hormone prolactin, which also has a libido-dampening effect, are at an all-time high.

✤ Lactational amenorrhea (the cessation of your menstrual period during lactation) keeps estrogen levels extremely low. Decreased estrogen levels may result in a significant reduction in vaginal lubrication and/or a thinning of vaginal walls, which can contribute to discomfort, soreness, and decreased pleasure. Once ovulation resumes, estrogen and androgen levels climb, bolstering your libido and making you juicy again. (See the next chapter for a more in-depth discussion of breastfeeding and sexual response.)

✤ Engorgement of your breasts may cause discomfort.

✤ Guilt—the old "you're a mother now" syndrome—can put a real damper on your sex drive. Sex is a necessity, not a self-ish indulgence. Pooh-pooh the notion that there's nobility in total self-sacrifice!

✤ The decreased intensity of postpregnancy orgasms can be frustrating.

✤ A traumatic delivery may require a significant emotional and physical recovery period for both partners.

✤ Some women develop thyroiditis or postpartum depression, both of which result in rapidly declining sex drive.

✤ The mother may be avoiding dealing with body image issues by not allowing herself to get sexy.

Be patient with yourself and your progress. Allison says, "I had an episiotomy and third-degree tear. It took me a long time to recover from it. I think I must've waited at least two months. Sex was pretty uncomfortable for a while. Too, I think everyone needs to be aware of what sex feels like when you're breastfeeding. It can feel like shards of glass because the lack of estrogen creates a lack of natural lube."

If you're not feeling up for a romp in the months following childbirth, know that you're not alone. This is a very normal response for a number of Hot Mamas, especially those who are breastfeeding. Your hormones are readjusting themselves, and the changes in your body are just temporary. You should be back on top of your game in no time.

In the meantime, alternative methods of experiencing physical intimacy may be easier, more appropriate, and less exhausting. For example, committing to a mere sixty seconds of pleasurable and/or nurturing touch each day will do wonders for both of you. Activities such as cuddling, shoulder and foot rubs, or simply looking deeply into each other's eyes for several seconds leading up to a passionate kiss can keep you connected during this transition phase. It is important that neither of you put an exaggerated amount of pressure on yourselves over this situation. Do not take a lack of sex personally, and practice patience with each other and yourselves.

Hot Mama, talk to your lover about what is going on with your body, factors impacting your sex drive, and what you're capable of doing. Partners are often hoping for some insight because they

HOW YOU CAN HELP HER

You can help alleviate the negative aspects of new motherhood for your partner. The issues a postpartum woman faces that contribute to her lack of libido include confinement, a lack of uninterrupted time and freedom to pursue personal interests, little or no social life, needing a break from the demands of the child, an inability to control and define the use of her time, loss of confidence, and difficulties coping with an infant's feeding and sleeping patterns. Partners can help mothers out by babysitting, which will give her some time to reconnect with herself, especially her sensual self, or, better still, by having a babysitter step in for even just an hour or two so the couple can have adult time, either together or apart. Sometimes she will need her lover to take the initiative in arranging some alone time for her, especially if she feels guilty about giving herself time away from the baby.

[for partners]

have lots of concerns and questions that may go unaddressed. Tom, a thirty-one-year-old criminologist, is thankful for the extra steps his wife took to communicate with him during her pregnancy and postbirth:

My wife's taking the initiative to talk about things was useful for me, because there were points when I was uncomfortable, like with breast milk. I didn't know how I was supposed to react. Her just asking me, "Are you not comfortable with this?" in the long run made things much easier. It's happening, so try not to pretend that it's not. From a guy's perspective, I really appreciate that she's carrying the majority of the burden of pregnancy. There are places, though, where a woman can take on more responsibility; the changes in her sexual feelings are in her court. So it's helpful not to treat it as some mystical event, but to have a discussion and allow him to try to understand her experiences. Guys don't want to imply that anything is problematic, but this is often what comes across when he asks questions while trying to figure things out, for example, about weight gain and how that feels. He needs the information from her to help make things better.

🐎 Getting Back into the Saddle

When you can and when you should have sex after childbirth are often two very different things. Depending upon whether you've undergone a C-section, an episiotomy, or severe tearing, you may need to wait a bit longer before resuming any sort of sex play. And the phenomenon of postbirth bleeding may be off-putting to some couples. Most childbirth practitioners, including Dr. Meulenberg, suggest that you wait at least four to six weeks before having intercourse. "I make all my patients wait until after their postpartum visit at six weeks," she says. "We check their perineum if they delivered vaginally to be sure that it healed well. Also, they should have their first period around that time [unless they're breast-feeding exclusively]. It does happen that some women come into the six-week visit pregnant again. That doesn't give their body any time to heal and can cause problems. The six-week visit is when we talk about family planning and birth control, so it is best just to hold off until then."

Here's Danielle:

Cravings for intimate and sensual touch returned in fits and starts for me. We indulged in some gentle petting, and we attempted penetration. But our sexual relationship did not resume in earnest until somewhere around seven weeks postbirth. When it happened, it was like losing my virginity all over again. As new parents, we were both different peo-ple. My vagina was a foreign land begging to be discovered. I had no idea what to expect. Rediscovering and reinventing my sexual self was a tearful and tender experience. Fortu-nately, thanks to Kegels and other pelvic exercises, my part-ner reported that it was like making love to a virgin. I was relieved. My secret fear that my vagina had been stretched too far to give pleasure was unfounded.

Allison is another woman who found sex to be better after childbirth: "My sex life improved after I had my son. My archi-tecture down there changed for the better. I noticed it about four months later, and I was really surprised since I was not always good at remembering to do my Kegels. I have read that one's vaginal walls change, so I'm not sure what helped me feel tighter."

When you take lovers' emotions into consideration, knowing when is the right time to resume lovemaking can become more complex. Exhaustion and crazy schedules aside, lovers may feel a bit overwhelmed about reconnecting sexually. Partners may harbor some of the typical misconceptions about postbirth intimacy. With both partners feeling a bit high strung, it is important to be gentle, respectful, and straight up with one another. Invite discussions, validate feelings, and share your hopes and concerns about what is to come. Postbirth sex can be intense and amazing, bringing you together like two young lovers exploring each other's body and touch for the first time. Taking things slowly, lovingly, and lightheartedly, with an open and adventuresome attitude, is key to becoming sexually intimate again. The other key is that you, Hot Mama, feel totally up for it.

Take your time rediscovering your pre-preggie sexual self. You may want to start with oral and manual pleasuring and work your way up to intercourse slowly, building the anticipation. Become brand-new lovers all over again. And when you're ready to "go all the way," start with easier positions that allow for slower, more sensual sex, like the side-by-side variations we covered in Chapter 3. Realize that you can do everything you could do before you became pregnant. Some activities may be less comfortable than others for now, but that will change soon enough. Pace yourself, and we're quite certain that you'll be your good ol' Hot Mama sexy self in no time.

🍀 What's Normal?

If you're curious about what is typical for other couples, studies have found that most start engaging in noncoital sexual contact about two to five weeks after childbirth, usually before intercourse has resumed. Intercourse, on average, is resumed six to eight weeks after birth in Europe and the United States. Before the sixth week postpartum, only 9–17 percent of couples are having sexual intercourse. This is a great time to share your shower or bath ritual with your partner. Lathering and touching each other can refresh your sense memory and start the slow-burn buildup to outright sexual longing.

By three months postpartum, nearly all couples have resumed having sexual intercourse. Shockingly, however, studies demonstrate that more men than women tend to be sexually disinterested at this point (maybe the only time men are actually lagging behind women in sexual desire). Many postpartum couples experience sexual difficulties overall, particularly lowered sexual desire and dyspareunia (painful intercourse), which brings us to the next saddening stat: Relationship satisfaction usually hits an all-time low during this period. Most couples claim moderate satisfaction within the first trimester postpartum, followed by significantly lower levels of relationship satisfaction well into the first year following childbirth.

A separate study of 570 women found that most women were equal in terms of when they recommenced sexual activity after childbirth, with one exception. Those who had cesareans generally resumed intercourse somewhat earlier. Something that frequently causes women with cesareans to wait a bit longer, though, is that they experience a sensation during early postpartum sex that the scar is about to burst open. Don't worry—as long as you're healed enough to avoid ripped stitches or excruciating pain, it won't. Avoid putting weight on the scar for several weeks after your foray back into sex play. And always get your doc's green light first.

We'll leave you with one more statistic, Hot Mama, and this one should be an encouraging one. There is a direct correlation between those couples reporting higher relationship satisfaction and those reporting greater frequency of sexual intercourse and less loss of sexual desire. If that's not incentive enough to shag, we don't know what is!

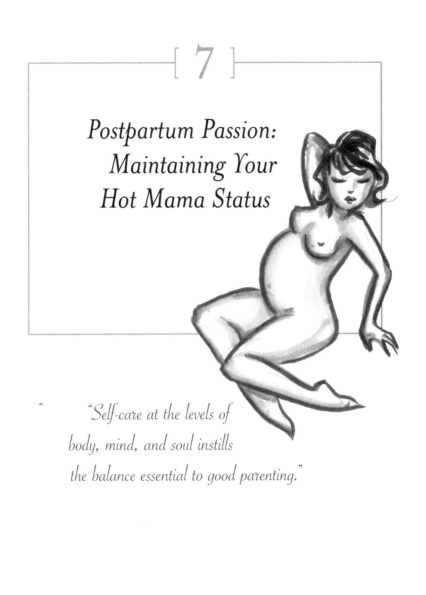

[7]

Postpartum Passion: Maintaining Your Hot Mama Status

"Self-care at the levels of body, mind, and soul instills the balance essential to good parenting."

*W*e could devote an entire book to everything couples need to know in order to maintain a hot sex life for the next eighteen-plus years. But we'll limit our focus here to getting you back into top-notch Hot Mama shape, because there are many factors that can impact how much intimacy you and your sweetheart will enjoy in the next year. As you evolve into motherhood it is important to recognize how this unique time can serve you, your relationship, and your sex life. You now have the opportunity—the perfect excuse—to reevaluate, reconceptualize, and redefine intimacy in your relationship. Regardless of how you see yourself in terms of your sexuality, use this chance to explore all the new and different ways you might share intimate, loving moments with your partner. You may actually enjoy a markedly improved sex life as a result.

In this chapter we'll address the major factors that could affect your game beyond the early-postpartum period covered in Chapter 6. With a little bit of awareness, and a handful of practical pointers, you should be feeling like your pre-preggie Hot Mama self in no time!

☙ Breastfeeding and Sexual Response

The breast—it's beautiful, it's erotic, it's a source of amazing pleasure. And for many of you, it's your baby's first "bottle." While breastfeeding a child is one of the most spectacular events a human being can ever experience, this gift may require a small trade-off for some of you. In study after study, breastfeeding is strongly correlated with reduced sexual desire in women and reduced frequency of intercourse in the early period after childbirth. One study in particular found that women who breastfed showed significantly less sexual activity and less sexual satisfaction than those who did not. Most of the women we interviewed reported reduced sexual satisfaction and sex drive as they wrestled simultaneously with feelings of guilt, shame, or being overwhelmed. Those who addressed these issues in discussions with their partner, or who simply let them go, seemed to enjoy a healthy postbirth rebound, almost as readily as their formula-feeding counterparts. And once breastfeeding has ceased, some women report experiencing orgasms that are more intense than ever, even trumping the intensified climaxes experienced during pregnancy.

It is extremely important to note that it is perfectly normal and natural for a mother to become aroused during breastfeeding. Strong surges of oxytocin released into your bloodstream during feedings, coupled with uterine contractions corresponding with your baby's suckling, can cause significant arousal. At least one-third to one-half of women surveyed feel that breastfeeding is an erotic experience, reporting *faire l'amour* with each feeding. Others admit to engaging in masturbation or sex in the moments after baby's done feeding. A minority of women actually climax during feedings. For shame? Hardly! Your nipples are an erogenous zone and this is part of a natural sexual response cycle. Some women are simply more sensitive than others, and that's nothing to be ashamed of. In fact, it's a bonus that other women may feel jealous of.

You can employ this oxytocin surge for your own dirty dealings. It'll do a world of good for your partnership and the rebounding of your sexuality. Harness the sensual feelings and the glowing, energetic love awakened during breastfeeding. Accumulate sensual energy in your lower abdomen while you're nursing your babe, and keep it ripe and ready for your lover later. Present your sexed-up self to your partner and revel in the sexy fun that results. Danielle did, with impressive results. Contrary to many of her girlfriends, who reported feeling guilty about their sexual feelings while breastfeeding, Danielle felt sensually awakened during the act of providing nourishment to her child. Trust us—it works! Mother Nature knew what she was doing. Many of us have simply forgotten how to listen.

Yet another joy of breastfeeding is your new squirt potential. If and when you have sex, your nipples may ejaculate milk during climax. This is an experience the lovely Julienne likes to retell: "My partner and I found ourselves in hysterics as my climax sprayed him with warm milk during one of our romps. 'Mama, you're lactating all over me!' he giggled. While a bit embarrassing at first, it was a bonding moment that has turned into a fond memory. He wasn't grossed out or disgusted, rather he was amused and strangely aroused. His casual and loving reaction lent itself to increased confidence in my sexual prowess and a decrease in my self-consciousness."

Another instance of breast-milk erotica found a lover trying to catch the squirting milk in his mouth as his Hot Mama had one of the most intense orgasms of her life. Amy, a twenty-seven-year-old Hot Mama from Los Angeles, recalls, "In the early days of weaning my son, my partner would nurse away some of the pain of engorgement. One particularly intense female-dominant sexcapade found my nipples squirting the wall directly above his head. It was so hot to look down and see his mouth opened in anticipation trying to catch the warm spray. I believe it may be the closest feeling to male ejaculation I've ever had the pleasure of experiencing. I've never felt more womanly and empowered!"

An interesting phenomenon in same-sex partnerships is the possibility of coincidental lactation at any time during the pregnancy. The nonpregnant partner may experience lactation in tandem with her Hot Mama, as thirty-five-year-old film producer Natasha describes: "Meghan, who is premenopausal, actually began lactating with me during the fourth month of our pregnancy. It was hysterical to go from quitting our periods for a long time, to sharing the breastfeeding experience, to adding milk to our sex play. Yummy fun!" An early appearance of milk in a pregnant woman is more anomaly than norm, but you can see how the hormonal synergy shared by female partners can have far-reaching implications similar to the couvade syndrome described in Chapter 3.

As mentioned in the last chapter, breastfeeding suppresses estrogen production from the ovaries, which results in decreased vaginal lubrication, even when you are sexually stimulated. If you fancy being intimate, you'll likely need to use saliva or a lubricant to counter the dryness. Danielle and her lover used K-Y Warming Jelly and Kama Sutra oils and loved them. Astroglide

---

WHAT'S GOING ON WITH YOUR PARTNER

Your partner may be turned off or aroused by the milk spouting from your nipples. If breast milk turns either of you off, schedule sex after a feeding or pumping. Many partners feel neglect when babe's on the boob 24/7, which is especially an issue with multiple births. So be sure to stroke your partner's ego with compliments, acknowledgement, and touch. Express your love and appreciation for him or her. Words may seem trite, but they really help to maintain lovers' emotional connection.

——————[**for hot mamas**]——————

---

is another great (though more costly) option; it tends to be more slippery than other lubricants.

Finally, another issue for a breastfeeding mother is that of feeling overtouched. Having constant physical contact with another human can be draining, comforting, or stimulating—depending on the day, the mindset, and the frequency. This can affect your desire for intimate touch with your partner, and it's one more important reason to keep the lines of communication open.

☙ Postpartum Birth Control (Yep, You Still Have to Worry)

When you start having sex again, birth control is an important consideration, even if you are breastfeeding. Most women will resume a regular menstrual cycle within six weeks of childbirth, although women who breastfeed exclusively have a natural period of lactational amenorrhea (LAM), during which there is no menstrual cycle for six months to a year. While breastfeeding does act as a contraceptive to a certain extent, it is not 100 percent reliable, especially after the appearance of your first menses. LAM is actually proven to be as effective as a number of commercial methods for longer than six months, provided the mother does not supplement feedings with formula *at all*. This means regular pumping and feeding at night—all night, every night. Still, Dr. Meulenberg warns not to be overly dependent on LAM for contraception. "I would never recommend relying on LAM for birth control since the failure rate is pretty high," she says. "There are other methods that are effective, such as progesterone-only OCPs [oral contraceptives], Depo Provera, IUDs, and condoms."

Ninety percent of couples use contraceptives postpartum, mostly the pill or condoms. Using birth control you trust and feel comfortable with is very important to help ease you through the sexual reattunement phase; plus, you'll more readily enjoy a higher degree of sexual satisfaction than if you were wavering. Many doctors swear by IUDs, which can be inserted soon after the birth while the cervix is still malleable, making installation less dramatic than at other times in a woman's life. Here's Dr. Meulenberg: "I *love* IUDs. I feel that they are great forms of birth control both for young professional women who can't worry about birth control but don't want children for a long time, and for women who think they are done with childbearing but are not ready for a tubal ligation. IUDs are just as effective as a tubal, last for five to ten years, and are reversible [unlike tubals]. Women who have them don't even know they are there. They are very small and can be easily inserted and removed by the OB-GYN in the office. I strongly recommend IUDs to all my patients."

Most IUDs are a nonhormonal contraceptive, so many nursing mothers feel the most comfortable with this method. Still, many women freak out at the thought of having a device implanted in their cervical region for up to ten years. If you feel at all squeamish about an IUD and don't think you'll get past it, please, do your sex life a favor and opt for a different method.

🦜 Postpartum Depression

Contending with postpartum depression can make it enormously difficult, if not impossible, to be intimate with your partner. A 2003 study found that women with postpartum depression were less likely to have resumed intercourse by the sixth month and were far likelier to suffer from sexual problems when they finally did. Watch yourself or have someone else to check in with if you suspect your malaise may be more than just a passing phase. And don't be afraid to seek out a mental-health counselor or therapist to help you deal with this most difficult situation.

🦜 Three's Company?

For couples who opt to have their newborn sleep in the master bedroom or in bed with them, having the baby in such close vicinity can be a bit unnerving when it comes to sex. With Mama

HOW YOU CAN HELP HER

Regular comments from you like, "Sexy mama," "Oooh, you're so sexy," or "You're sexier than ever" can work wonders to help your Hot Mama get past any issues she might have concerning body image and motherhood. Your well-timed compliments can boost both her ego and spirits. She has given birth to your child and needs to be hailed as the goddess mother she is. Given the subtle and not-so-subtle changes her body has undergone—for example, carrying extra tissue around her lower abs—hearing positive statements from her lover is of paramount importance. Julienne explains, "While I loved my body, I felt shy around my husband at first, fearing that he would no longer want me with the more ample curves. Never again could I be that hot young thing! I was a mother, and no amount of working out or dieting would change the fact that I perceived my body differently, with more deference, but with a little bit of fear as well. I was worried that he would, as the media would have you believe all men would, secretly fantasize and pine away over twenty-year-old, air-brushed gals while we were in the throes of passion. I feared he'd see me in my underthings, postpregnancy 'imperfections' and all, only to view our culture's sexual ideals five minutes later on the TV in our living room. It's not easy reentering a society which objectifies women in such overt and subtle ways."

{ *for partners* }

and Papa aware of the little one's every noise—every breath, sniff, or cough—anxiety may impinge on sex play. Know that babies have a very limited awareness about what's going on when parents make love, as renowned pediatrician Dr. William Sears assures couples in his books.

Cosleeping is an important, personal decision for every family to sort through. Talk to each other honestly about how the baby's close presence may impact your sex life. Having the baby right there could be a turn-off, or it could be more disconcerting for the babe to be in its own room during your lovemaking. For many couples, having the babe sleep close by for up to a year is no big deal, while for others that time period feels absolutely eternal.

༃ Pencil Me In: Making Sex a Priority

Amid the chaos and exhaustion following a new arrival, partners often find themselves with nothing left for one another. Research from 1990 that tracked ninety-seven couples following the birth of their first child found that while both partners reported a peak in their marital adjustment at one month postpartum, both also reported a significant decline in this area at six months postbirth.

You know that it is important to hug, kiss, cuddle, and connect in these delicate, postbirth days when really *seeing* your lover can be difficult. Maintaining a conscious awareness of one another is vital throughout this entire phase of your partnership, from conception beyond birth. And it is totally up to the two of you how you want to do this. Still, for your sex life to continue, you must make it a priority. You must focus on creating time and space for your lover, or having children may cost you your partnership. That is never a good outcome, so let's get to work. Get out your schedule books and, based on your baby's sleep schedule, actually plan for sex. Write it down, and don't let anything get in the way of your plans. Set aside a couple of evenings per month when you will have a babysitter. Whether it's your mom, your partner's sister, your best friend, or another new mom, there are probably plenty of people in your circle who would love to spend a couple of hours with your little one. Take advantage of friends' and relatives' offers to help. Taking the time to nurture your relationship for a few hours each month doesn't make you a "bad mother," especially when you consider that your little one owns you for most hours of every day.

❦ Baby's Sex Radar

One huge issue for new parents is that baby often seems to have a sex radar. Even when the timing is perfect and the little cherub is sound asleep, as soon as the action gets hot and heavy little cries for attention penetrate the love magic. Many mothers are convinced that the mother–child connection triggers some survival-related alarm in the infant's sixth sense, alerting him or her that mommy's attention is suddenly being channeled elsewhere. Baby's instincts just aren't cool with sharing!

Now, it's likely that it only *seems* as though every time you're about to do the nasty, the nasty wails begin. Either way, cries that break the romantic spell can spell sexual disaster. Many parents say that ignoring the crying works just fine. Danielle let her newborn scream along to the moans of adult ecstasy. But others may find this irritant simply too much to shut out. The stress response to a baby's crying is hard-wired into all adults to some degree, which may render sexual antics absolutely unthinkable when baby's unhappy. Consider this: An orgasm can do wonders to relieve the stress a mother feels in response to her child's crying. The increased tension she's been carrying may even intensify her climax. Furthermore, the baby is not going to die if you let him or her cry for a few extra moments while you finish your business. Although it's important to be attentive to your baby, overly doting on him or her by rushing to answer every wail is not going to do either of you any good in the long run, as many developmental psychologists will tell you.

Given the challenges of sexing it up with a new baby in the house, we (once again) strongly recommend letting someone take care of the baby as soon as you're comfortable doing so, even if only for an hour or two. Even if you're madly committed to your breastfeeding routine, with no intention of pumping, you will want to figure out a time between feedings to let another adult keep your babe so you can tend to your partner and vice versa. Don't let your relationship break down due to your decision to breastfeed. Your partner, who is also a new parent, is likely to be experiencing emotional turmoil, including fear of the unknown, fear of failing to be a good parent, stress over finances, stress about hurting you, stress over the state of your vagina, and so on. It's vital for you to offer your partner your one-on-one, baby-free attention

> ### How You Can Help Her
>
> *Let her know that you're there for her, willing to take care of the baby, and that you understand the difficulties she's dealing with. Furthermore, don't wait to be asked to do something—just do it!*
>
> ─┤ **for partners** ├─

from time to time. You must regularly connect with one another or risk living parallel lives without much sexual, sensual, or intimate gratification.

⚘ Other Hot Mama Postpartum Tips

Below is a grab bag of easy-to-implement suggestions for staying in Hot Mama form. The items in the list range from ways to keep your energy level up to strategies for staying attractive to your partner. The more you remain on top of your game, fighting all the little things that can make you feel—and look—haggard, the more game play you'll see with your lover.

- ❖ Make breastfeeding stress-free. Have everything you need in one place, for example, your phone, magazines, snacks, the TV remote, paper towels, footstool, baby blanket, headrest —whatever you can think of that will make breastfeeding easier and more comfortable.

- ❖ Nap when your little one does. You need your energy to be a Hot Mama!

❖ Walk. Connect to the world around you, move your body, and feel better.

❖ Join a Hot Mama support group. A new mother's group is a safe place to share all of your joys and gripes, to feel validated and understood, and to get information.

❖ Keep a list of good babysitters handy so that you can steal away at a moment's notice, even if just for a solo trip to the grocery store.

❖ Make a list of priorities, and abide by it. Enlist your partner's help in drafting the list so that everyone knows what's going on when the socks start piling up. (That's when you say, "Oh honey, that's *last* on my list!")

❖ Ask for help. Say yes to any offer of shopping, cleaning, cooking, or child supervision.

❖ Take care of yourself. Visit the hair salon. Buy feel-good clothes for your transition phase. Exercise. Reread Chapter 5.

❖ Join a gym or diet club if extra weight is posing a challenge.

❖ Be nice to your partner—no snapping!

Self-care at the levels of body, mind, and soul instills the balance essential to good parenting. Both during and after pregnancy, all the Hot Mamas we interviewed noted the importance of realizing that while motherhood will enhance your life in unimaginable ways, if should not become your *entire* life. Continuing to dream and create is vital to raising well-adjusted children and maintaining your autonomy as parenthood threatens to take over every aspect of your self.

If you require an incentive to spend some of your precious energy taking care of yourself and your needs, think back to any of your peers whose parents tried to live vicariously through them or who burdened them with the feeling that the kids had somehow impeded the parents' lives. People waste years and tears recovering from those sorts of dynamics with their parents, so you may want to reconsider your vision of yourself as the self-sacrificing, "perfect" mom. Hot Mamas know that autonomy and breathing room translate directly into increased intimacy with their partners and greater satisfaction with their lives.

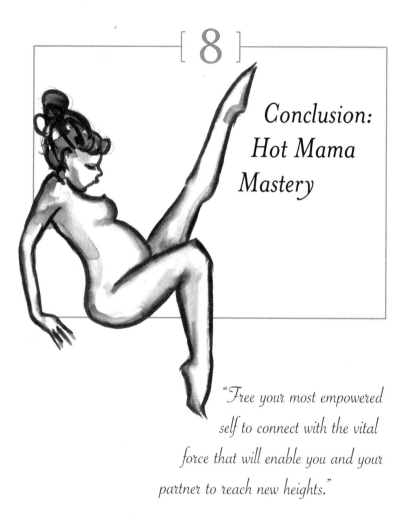

[8]

Conclusion: Hot Mama Mastery

"Free your most empowered self to connect with the vital force that will enable you and your partner to reach new heights."

*W*hile conclusions are often meant to wrap things up, we hope that this send off marks the start of your sensual journey into the Hot Mama lifestyle. You've done an amazing job embracing and owning your Hot Mama nature. You've shirked convention and taken up the cause to inspire would-be Hot Mamas everywhere. You've joined the Hot Mama campaign and learned to raise your Hot Mama hot factor to its fullest. And we're just getting warmed up!

We urge you to continue cultivating your own sensual nature, delving deeper into the throes of your sexual being and becoming the beacon of sensuality aspiring Hot Mamas can look up to. By forging your own path, you will teach other women that loving your body, your pregnancy, your sensuality is the cornerstone of an orgasmic pregnancy and postpartum. That's right, Hot Mama, your sensual mastery can actually change the lives of others! We think that in and of itself is cause enough to join us in our quest to awaken the Hot Mama in women everywhere.

So remember to stay fully in your body and fully in tune with its rhythms every day. Hot Mamas never let a day go by in which they do not acknowledge and honor their sensuality in at least some small way. Learn to be gentle with yourself, your partner, your schedule, your chores... You really can have it all, including a super sex life. It's all a matter of perspective, and we hope that the Hot Mama mantras and lessons herein have inspired you to strive for your most orgasmic experiences to date.

Even if you're a slow-starting Hot Mama, place sensual pleasures at the top of your priority list. Give yourself permission to enjoy some well-deserved fun. Treat yourself with kindness, respect, and love, and allow your partner the space to err and explore next to you. Be vulnerable. Be raw. Be real. It's your Hot Mama prerogative to design your sexy self in whatever way you see fit, no apologies!

Thank you, Hot Mama, for allowing us to be part of this most important and precious time in your life. We hope you've been inspired to the best orgasms of your life—and that there are many more to come! We hope that you and your lover have embarked on a ceaseless journey to explore new delights and adventures, and that you find yourselves increasingly fulfilled and better connected than ever.

Congratulations, Hot Mama! You are well on your way to unleashing your fullest sexual potential and becoming a true sexual master. We wish you and your new family all the best of life, love, and orgasm!

XX,
Your Hot Mama mentors,
Danielle and Yvonne

Female External and Internal Sexual Anatomy

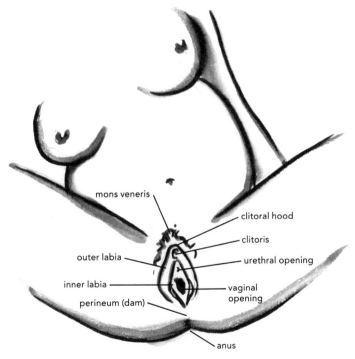

FIGURE A.1
The female external sexual anatomy

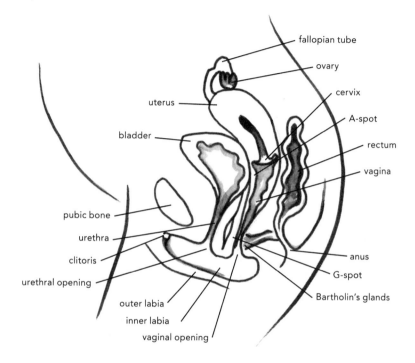

FIGURE A.2
The female internal sexual anatomy

References

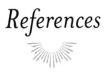

Adams, W. J. (1988). Sexuality and happiness ratings of husbands and wives in relation to first and second pregnancy. *Journal of Family Psychology*, 2, 67–81.

Bartellas, E., Crane, J. M., Daley, M., Bennett, K. A., and Hutchens, D. (2000). Sexuality and sexual activity in pregnancy. *British Journal of Obstetrics and Gynecology*, 107 (8), 964–968.

Byrd, J. E., Hyde, J. S., DeLamater, J. D., and Plant, E. A. (1998). Sexuality during pregnancy and the year postpartum. *Journal of Family Practice*, 47 (4), 305–308.

Fisher, C., Cohen, H. D., Schiavi, R. C., Davis, D., Furman, B., Ward, K., Edwards, A., and Cunningham, J. (1983). Patterns of female sexual arousal during sleep and waking: Vaginal thermo-conductance studies. *Archives of Sexual Behavior*, 12, 97–122.

Friedman, N. A. (1999). The experience of pregnancy for lesbian couples. *Dissertation Abstracts International*, 59 (8-B), 4536.

Ganem, M. B. (1992). *La Sexualité du Couple Pendant la Grossesse: Guide Pratique* [The Couple's Sexuality During Pregnancy: A Practical Guide]. Paris: Éditions Filipacchi.

Gokyildiz, S., and Beji, N. K. (2005). The effects of pregnancy on sexual life. *Journal of Sex and Marital Therapy*, 31 (3), 201–215.

Gottman, J., and Silver, N. (2000). *The Seven Principles for Making Marriage Work*. New York: Three Rivers Press.

Gray, R. H., Li, X., Kigozi, G., et al. (2005). Increased risk of incident HIV during pregnancy in Rakai, Uganda: A prospective study. *Lancet*, 366 (9492), 1182–1188.

Heinig, L., and Enfer, A. (1988). Schwangerschaft und partnerschaft. *Report Psychologie*, 13, 56–59.

Hyde, J. S., DeLamater, J. D., and Hewitt, E. C. (1998). Sexuality and the dual-earner couple: Multiple roles and sexual functioning. *Journal of Family Psychology*, 12, 354–368.

Koelman, C. A., Coumans, A. B., Nijman, H. W., Doxiadis, I. I., Dekker, G. A., and Claas, F. H. (2000). Correlation between oral sex and a low incidence of preeclampsia: A role for soluble HLA in seminal fluid? *Journal of Reproductive Immunology*, 46 (2), 155–166.

Latifses, V. (2004). Teaching expectant fathers to massage their partners: An exploration of fetal attachment behaviors, anxiety, and marital adjustment in fathers. *Dissertation Abstracts International*, 64 (12-B), 6332.

Masters, W. H., and Johnson, V. (1996). *Human Sexual Response*. Boston: Little, Brown.

Morof, D., Barrett, G., Peacock, J., Victor, C. R., and Manyonda, I. (2003). Postnatal depression and sexual health after childbirth. *Obstetrics and Gynecology*, 102 (6), 1318–1325.

MUNMED. (1999, Summer). *Pregnancy and Sex*. Retrieved May 7, 2007, from http://www.med.mun.ca/munmed/112/bartella.htm.

Oken, E., Taveras, E., Popoola, F., Rich-Edward, J., and Gilman, M. (2007). Television, walking, and diet: Associations with postpartum weight retention. *American Journal of Preventive Medicine*, 32 (4).

Pasini, W. (1980). *Psychosomatik in Sexualitat und Gynakologie*. Stuttgart: Hippokrates.

Sayle, A. E., Savitz, D. A., Thorp, J. M., Hertz-Picciotto, I., and Wilcox, A. J. (2001). Sexual activity during late pregnancy and risk of preterm delivery. *Obstetrics and Gynecology*, 97 (2), 283–289.

Snowden, L. R., Schott, T. L., Awalt, S. J., and Gillis-Knox, J. (1988). Marital satisfaction in pregnancy: Stability and change. *Journal of Marriage and the Family*, 50, 325–333.

Tan, P. C., Andi, A., Azmi, N., and Noraihan, M. N. (2006). Effect of coitus at term on length of gestation, induction of labor, and mode of delivery. *Journal of Obstetrics and Gynecology*, 108, 134–140.

Von Sydow, K. (1999). Sexuality during pregnancy and after childbirth: A metacontent analysis of 59 studies. *Journal of Psychosomatic Research, 47* (1), 27–49.

Wallace, P. M., and Gotlib, I. H. (1990). Marital adjustment during the transition to parenthood: Stability and predictors of change. *Journal of Marriage and the Family, 52* (1), 21–29.

Whipple, B., Ogden, G., and Komisaruk, B. R. (1992). Physiological correlates of imagery-induced orgasm in women. *Archives of Sexual Behavior, 21* (2), 121–133.

Wilkerson, N. N., and Shrock, P. (2000). Sexuality in the perinatal period. In S. S. Humenick and F. H. Nichols (eds.), *Childbirth Education: Practice, Research, and Theory* (pp. 48–65). Philadelphia: W. B. Saunders Co.

Willey, V.L. (2003). Changes in sexuality during pregnancy. *Dissertation Abstracts International, 63* (10-B), 4930.

Resources

Acupressure Points

Gach, Michael Reed. *Acupressure for Lovers*. New York: Bantam Books, 1997.

Sollars, David W. *The Complete Idiot's Guide to Acupuncture and Acupressure*. New York: Penguin, 2000.

www.childbirthsolutions.com/articles/birth/acupressure/index.php

Anal Sex

Taormino, Tristan. *The Ultimate Guide to Anal Sex for Women*, 2nd ed. San Francisco, CA: Cleis Press, 2006.

http://parenting.ivillage.com/pregnancy/psex/0,,midwife_3pjq,00.html

Breathing/Meditation

www.healthandyoga.com/html/pbreath.html

Essential Oils

www.mountainroseherbs.com

www.youngliving.com

Fantasy

Blue, Violet. *Taboo: Forbidden Fantasies for Couples*. San Francisco, CA: Cleis Press, 2004.

Fashion During Pregnancy

www.apeainapod.com

www.babiesnbellies.com

www.bellybasics.com

www.figure8maternity.com

www.glamourmom.com

www.japaneseweekend.com
www.noppies.com
www.lizlange.com
www.rockstarmoms.com
www.unbuttonedmaternity.com

Female Ejaculation

Sundahl, Deborah. *Female Ejaculation and the G-Spot.* Alameda, CA: Hunter House Publishers, 2003.

Fitness and Nutrition

www.epicurious.com
www.pregnancywithoutpounds.com

General Pregnancy

www.babyzone.com
http://expectantmothersguide.com/library/pittsburgh/sex.htm

G-Spot

Whipple, Beverly, John D. Perry, and Alice Khan Ladas. *The G-Spot and Other Discoveries about Human Sexuality.* New York: Owl Books, 2004.

Winks, Cathy. *The Good Vibrations Guide: The G-Spot.* San Francisco, CA: Down There Press, 1998.

Kama Sutra

Link, Al, and Pala Copeland. *The Supercharged Kama Sutra.* New York: Alpha Books, 2006.

Wikoff, Johanna, and Deborah S. Romaine. *The Complete Idiot's Guide to the Kama Sutra.* New York: Alpha Books, 2004.

Lingerie

www.agentprovocateur.com
www.apeainapod.com
www.bellamaterna.com

www.gap.com
www.lrsmaternity.com

Massage

Inkeles, Gordon. *Massage for a Peaceful Pregnancy.* Bayside, CA: Arcata Arts, 2006.

http://pregnancytoday.com/reference/articles/prenatms.htm
www.pregopillow.com
www.rhythmmassagenyc.com

Masturbation

Dodson, Betty. *Sex for One.* New York: Harmony Books, 1996.

Oral Sex

http://pregnancy.about.com/cs/sexuality/a/pregsex_2.htm

Piercings

www.pregnancypiercings.com

Pregnant Porn

www.pregnanthoney.com/planet-preggo.html

Pregnancy Resource Books

Evans, Joel, and Robin Aronson. The Whole Pregnancy Handbook. New York: Gotham, 2005.

Ganem, Marc. *La Sexualité du Couple Pendant la Grossesse* [The Couple's Sexuality During Pregnancy]. Paris: Éditions Filipacchi, 1992.

Prenatal Yoga

www.healthandyoga.com/html/pbreath.html
www.pauladatkinson.com
www.prenatalyogadvd.com

Reflexology

Chia, Mantak, and William U. Wei. Sexual Reflexology. Rochester, NY: Destiny Books, 2003.

Kunz, Barbara, and Kevin Kunz. *Reflexology: Health at Your Fingertips.* New York: DK Publishing, 2003.

Sex Coaching

Sensual Fusion
www.sensualfusion.com

Sex Toys

Sensual Fusion Soirées
www.sensualfusionsoirees.com

Adam and Eve
www.adameve.com

Condomania
www.condomania.com

Eve's Garden
www.evesgarden.com

Good Vibrations (catalogs)
www.goodvibes.com

Intimate Gifts
www.intimategifts.com

Liberator Shapes
www.liberatorshapes.com

Toys in Babeland
www.babeland.com

Sexual Fitness

www.mygoals.com/categoryPages/pub-createGP-fromCategorySexSexual
Fitness.html

Sex Education and Information

Go Ask Alice!
www.goaskalice.columbia.edu
Columbia University's health-education website

San Francisco Sex Information
P.O. Box 881254
San Francisco CA 94188-1254
(877) 472-SFSI (7374)
(415) 989-7374
www.sfsi.org
Features frequently asked questions, weekly columns, and referrals

Sexuality Information and Education Council of the United States
(212) 819-0109
www.siecus.org
Nonprofit organization providing sex education programs and materials

Sexuality Source, Inc.
www.sexualitysource.com (or www.yvonnekfulbright.com)
Offers sex education and consulting services, free newsletter; is affiliated with
www.sensualfusion.com

Society for Human Sexuality
www.sexuality.org
Features information and articles on a variety of sex topics, as well as book,
video, and product reviews

Spanish Sexuality website
www.gentejoven.org.mx

WebMD
www.webmd.com

Sex Therapy

American Association of Sex Educators, Counselors, and Therapists

www.aasect.org

Sexual Pleasuring

Chalker, Rebecca. *The Clitoral Truth: The Secret World at Your Fingertips.* New York: Seven Stories Press, 2000.

Fulbright, Yvonne K. *The Hot Guide to Safer Sex.* Alameda, CA: Hunter House Publishers, 2003.

Fulbright, Yvonne K. *Touch Me There! A Hands-On Guide to Your Orgasmic Hot Spots.* Alameda, CA: Hunter House, 2007.

Keesling, Barbara. *Sexual Pleasure*, 2nd edition. Alameda, CA: Hunter House Publishers, 2005.

Index

More Hunter House Books

TOUCH ME THERE! A Hands-On Guide to Your Orgasmic Hot Spots
by Yvonne K. Fulbright, PhD

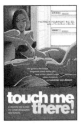

Fulbright teaches readers how to use fresh techniques, positions, and ideas for enhanced orgasmic experiences. She also illustrates — with pictures — how to find and awaken little-known erotic pleasure points that she has discovered through her study of tantric sex, yoga, acupressure, and reflexology.

240 pages ... 58 illus. ... Paperback $14.95

THE HOT GUIDE TO SAFER SEX
by Yvonne K. Fulbright, PhD

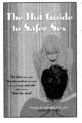

Tackling safer sex in a hip, entertaining tone, Yvonne explains how readers can lower their risk of getting an STD while improving the overall quality of their sexual experiences. Chapters include: "You Always Can in Fantasyland," "Horny & High: What Drugs Really Do to Your Sex Life," and "Making a Multi-Orgasmic Man."

352 pages ... 57 illus. ... Paperback $14.95

FEMALE EJACULATION & THE G-SPOT
by Deborah Sundahl

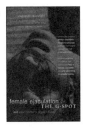

All women have a G-spot, which is a their prostate gland. It swells with blood when stimulated and can emit ejaculate fluid, usually during orgasm. This book describes exercises, techniques, and positions that help a woman ejaculate, and also shows men how to help their female partners to ejaculate.

240 pages ... 13 illus. ... Paperback $16.95

TANTRIC SEX FOR WOMEN: A Guide for Lesbian, Bi, Hetero and Solo Lovers
by Christa Schulte

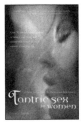

Christa Schulte introduces women to tantric methods for enhancing sexuality and spirituality. With over 50 exercises and games, rituals, meditations, and massage techniques, she helps women of every sexual orientation explore sensual potential, enrich relationships, and enjoy the small ecstasies of everyday life.

288 pages ... 18 illus. ... Paperback $16.95

More Hunter House Books

WOMEN'S SEXUAL PASSAGES:
Finding Pleasure and Intimacy at Every Stage of Life *by Elizabeth Davis*

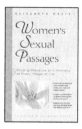

Davis unravels the mystery of how and why women's sexual desires change over their lifetime. She blends lessons on physicality, emotion, intuition, creativity, and spirituality with discussions of hormones and biological rhythms, menstruation and pregnancy, birth and child rearing.

288 pages ... 1 Illus. ... Paperback $15.95

RELIEVING PELVIC PAIN DURING AND AFTER PREGNANCY: How Women Can Heal Chronic Pelvic Instability *by Cecile Röst, PT*

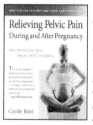

Pregnancy weakens the ligaments that keep the pelvic bones together, which can result in instability and pain that may last for weeks, even years. Cecile Röst, a physical therapist, has devised a simple treatment program that does not cause any pain, can be done at home or under supervision, and has a 90 percent success rate. In **Part One** she explains symmetry and stabilization exercises for the pelvis, and the best positions for sitting, lying, and other daily activities. **Part Two** is for care providers and gives background information about pelvic pain and advanced details of the therapy.

160 pages ... 139 illus. ... Paperback $16.95

NATURAL BIRTH CONTROL MADE SIMPLE *by Barbara Kass-Annese, RN, CNP, and Hal C. Danzer, MD*

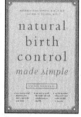

This book shows women how to chart their fertility signs to determine when they are infertile and can safely have intercourse without conceiving. These techniques can be used alone or combined with other methods of contraception. They are noninvasive, avoid the danger of toxic infection, inexpensive, and self-directed. With over 50 illustrations and charts and extensive resources.

192 pages ... 66 Illus. ... Paperback $13.95

Also available in a Spanish-language edition : **Simples Métodos de Control de la Natalidad**

208 pages ... 66 illus. ... Paperback $13.95